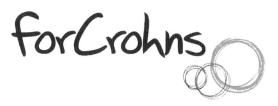

Presents

Book forCrohn's

Written by the Crohn's community for the Crohn's community

ISBN: 1500601691
ISBN 13: 9781500601690

Foreword

When I first started to suffer from Crohn's disease, I was just a child. It sounds silly, but as many of the people in this book point out, I didn't really realise how ill I was. As a child, you just think everyone feels the way you do.

It was the early 80s and little was known about Crohn's at the time. Endlessly, doctors said I was "just" anorexic or "just" depressed. Years of damage went unchecked and untreated until I was finally diagnosed at 16.

Even then, I only found out that I had Crohn's because an unsuspecting locum let it slip. I rushed home – there was no internet then – and found a book on my mum's bookshelf, a 1970s dictionary of illnesses and diseases, their signs and symptoms. I'll never forget what it said: "Crohn's is the condition of the overachiever, always striving for the next trophy. A period of rest, accepting that one is not superhuman, will often bring about a remission."

And so for years, I felt somehow to blame. All those years of being told it was "all in my head" crystallised in that short phrase.

I didn't know anyone else with Crohn's, my friends had no idea what it meant and my family could only watch helplessly as I got more and more unwell. No one around me lived a life like mine, no one knew how I felt or understood the challenges I faced.

Most frustratingly, I often found that those in the medical profession knew even less than I did. Worse, I often found that they were dismissive or judgmental. I seemed to spend more time fighting for treatment, acceptance or support than I did just trying to live with the increasingly distressing symptoms.

Happily, things are very different today. I've seen great strides in treatment and understanding. Now, whenever I say I have Crohn's, I'm told: "Oh, my sister/nephew/friend has that". Schools have information on dealing with sufferers, often just children when the disease takes hold, and there is a whole range of medications and treatments that can help.

However, serious illness of any kind can be isolating and confusing. Medical care is still often patchy or inadequate and there is often a lack of local support. This book is possibly the most important development I've seen in the 30 years I've spent fighting for a better understanding of IBD. The medical opinions are clear and easy to understand, but most importantly, sufferers of Crohn's tell their own stories and for many readers, I imagine it will be the first time they've seen their own lives, their own challenges, there in black and white on the page. That moment when you realise you're not alone, that others have the same strange symptom or side-effect as you do, can be incredibly powerful.

I believe passionately that knowledge brings solutions. If you understand why something happens and what causes it, you're just a step away from treating it. This book allows one Crohn's sufferer to talk to another, and when we talk, we find answers. So often the patient gets forgotten, but this book puts our shared experiences at the very centre of empowering us to be the best that we can be.

Sue Marsh has suffered from severe Crohn's disease for over 30 years. Happily married with two young boys, she writes about the challenges of living life with a serious long-term illness and set up the blog Diary of a Benefit Scrounger to campaign for better care and support. She writes about patient care and social security issues for the Guardian and other outlets, and regularly appears on our news bulletins discussing issues relating to health and welfare.

Contents

1. **Crohn's disease from the medics**   1

   The medical sections of Book forCrohn's have been written by a variety of clinicians. These are the people who see Crohn's disease every day; they diagnose it, treat it, operate on it and improve the lives of those who have it, so it makes sense to get the facts from them first! This section will give you all the basic information you need to get to grips with Crohn's disease.

2. **Crohn's disease from those with the condition**   15

   Book forCrohn's would not be complete without hearing from those who live with the condition every day. In this section, people with Crohn's disease give refreshingly honest and inspiring accounts of their experiences of living with the condition. Healthcare professionals have commented on these accounts to help explain some of the more technical parts but the stories have not been altered in content, so they include some of the myths and misunderstandings that so commonly surround Crohn's disease. The medics have instead pointed these out to highlight them and explain their origins. Sections:

Introduction

Although Crohn's disease can be a difficult condition to live with, it doesn't need to stand in the way of a fulfilling life.

The journey ahead may be a tough one, but we hope that our book will arm you with an insight into what to expect, and inspire you with accounts of how to live a full and happy life with Crohn's disease.

Everyone who has contributed to this book is living with Crohn's disease in some way or another. We are those with the condition, the parents, the children, the partners, the friends and the healthcare professionals who treat and research the disease. Whatever our relationship to the condition, we deal with Crohn's disease on a daily basis and understand exactly how it can affect everyday life; not just for the patient but for those around them. We understand how many questions there are to be answered and the scarcity of literature out there equipped to deal with them.

In short, this book is designed not only for the person with the condition but also for everyone around them. It contains all of the medical explanations you would want from a book about Crohn's disease, but most importantly, we have filled it with the personal accounts of people living with the condition. All of the accounts are refreshingly honest, showing both the good and bad times, and have been commented on by healthcare professionals – from dietitians, to surgeons and psychiatrists. We've included the practical as well as the emotional; whether it's tips on what to expect when having surgery or how Crohn's may affect your relationships – you will find it all here.

We think it's really important for those with Crohn's to be able to tell their story and invite you to share yours - www.forcrohns.org and help the community live beyond this book.

The team behind Book forCrohn's

forCrohns

forCrohns is the only UK volunteer-run charity solely dedicated to funding research into and raising awareness of Crohn's disease. Everyone on our committee either has Crohn's or has a close family member or friend with the condition, so you won't find a more passionate group of people determined to beat this disease.

forCrohns' mission is to fund research that helps those with the condition today and contributes to finding a cure for Crohn's disease in the future, while making more people in the UK aware of the disease and its symptoms.

For more information on forCrohns, to get involved with our events or find a Crohn's buddy, please visit www.forCrohns.org

We have deliberately kept the cost of Book forCrohn's as low as possible, to ensure it is accessible to the largest number of people. The small profit that is made from the sale of Book forCrohn's goes directly to fund research into Crohn's disease. If you would like to make a further donation to the charity, please visit our website for details.

The team behind Book forCrohn's

Most of the authors who contributed to Book forCrohn's are those with the condition, who kindly volunteered to share their story after being recruited through forCrohns events, social media and posters distributed around hospitals. There is also a team of medics who have explained their areas of expertise in layman's terms, and helped annotate the stories you'll find in each chapter.

The core team who brought the book together is comprised of the forCrohns trustees and co-founders, Tasha and Lisa; volunteer committee members, Sally and Phil W; and our medical expert, Phil T.

The motivation behind the project

Tasha Adley

During the last decade of co-running the forCrohns charity, I have seen the power of community support that has come from social networks such as Twitter and Facebook, but also the lack of depth to this information. Book forCrohn's seemed like a fantastic opportunity to replicate some of this community spirit and combine it with the medical expertise we are fortunate to have access to. As the daughter of someone with Crohn's disease, I also appreciate, on a personal level, the importance of a relatives section, which feels particularly unique to this book. In addition, the book has become particularly relevant to me as I have been going through the Crohn's diagnostic process as this project comes to completion. I hope that it is able to bring information and support to a huge number of people affected by Crohn's disease and is as useful to them as it has been to me.

Lisa Walker

Crohn's disease can feel like an overwhelming condition and certainly one that people don't instantly recognise or understand. I've been really excited to bring together a book that acts as a 'one stop shop' for those with Crohn's and their family to visit when they want an insight into the condition, a motivational tool or to feel like they are not alone. As co-founder of forCrohns, I am really proud of our achievement with this book and the support I hope it will offer many people.

Phil Walker

Through forCrohns, I have seen how Crohn's disease can impact people's lives, how daunting the experience can be and how important a person's support network can be. I wanted to be a part of creating something that could help people to better understand and cope with the disease, to let them know they're not alone in what they face and to give them hope for the future. If this book can inform and inspire just one person, then I will consider it a success, but obviously I hope it will be useful for many more.

Phil Tozer

Knowledge is power. Patients are always and understandably frightened about things they don't fully understand. Crohn's is a complex disease with many different options for treatment and a wide range of implications for those who suffer and their friends and families. I hope this book will help to give some power and control back to the patient and their supporters in their battle with Crohn's,

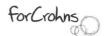

help them get the most from health care professionals striving to look after them and help them help themselves.

Sally Cooney

I was diagnosed with Crohn's eight years ago, at the age of 22. I have suffered severely over the years and have undergone five operations and numerous hospital stays. I decided to get involved with this book as I would have loved something similar when I was diagnosed. It can be a lonely time and I think you can take great comfort from reading people's experiences. It was of paramount importance to me to keep the book 'real' and not sugar-coat anything. I really hope that people find the medical information useful and the patient stories as inspirational as I have.

Healthcare Professionals

Phil Tozer

Phil is a surgical registrar whose research interest is fistula in Crohn's disease. He is part of the London surgical training program as a colorectal trainee. His research took place at St Mark's Hospital where he continues his research interest with the Fistula Research Unit.

Phil Smith

Phil is a gastroenterology registrar who not only has Crohn's disease, but has also done his PhD research in this area and is training to be an IBD specialist. Phil works in North East and Central London on his gastroenterology rotation and has worked within the British Society of Gastroenterology for the last few years developing educational projects for the consultants of the future.

Lucy Medcalf

Lucy has been an Inflammatory Bowel Disease Nurse Specialist since 2004 initially at UCLH now working at St George's Hospital in South-West London. She is keen to ensure that patients have access to information & encourages them by helping to run an evening support group every 3 months.

Ana Wilson

Ana is a consultant gastroenterologist at St Mark's Hospital with interests in colonoscopy and inflammatory bowel disease. Having completed her research degree at St Mark's Hospital, she is currently a co-investigator on numerous trials looking at new treatments for inflammatory bowel disease.

Warren Hyer

Warren is a paediatric gastroenterologist at St Mark's Hospital and has a strong clinical and research interest in IBD in children. He has published a number of scientific papers on various aspects of paediatric gastroenterology, and has gained experience in internationally-renowned units in Australia and Canada, in addition to St Mark's.

Alison Culkin

Alison is a research dietitian who has worked at St Mark's since 1998, completing her PhD in 2010. She is part of the nutrition team, providing enteral and parenteral nutrition to patients with intestinal failure, including those with inflammatory bowel disease.

Julian Stern

Julian completed his psychiatry and adult psychotherapy training at the Maudsley Hospital. For 17 years, he was the consultant psychiatrist in psychotherapy at St Mark's Hospital. He has a particular interest in working psychotherapeutically in a medical setting, both with staff members and with patients. He has published widely both in gastroenterology and psychiatry journals and books.

Illustrator: Alin Balaj

Dr Balaj worked in the UK between 2010 and 2013 at the QEII Hospital in Welwyn Garden City where he met Phil Tozer. The two have been friends ever since. Alin's artistic talents were immediately obvious to Phil and he kindly agreed to create the diagrams in this book as a free service to forCrohns. He has now returned to his home country of Romania where he practices in the County Emergency Clinical Hospital, Oradea, as a Specialist in General Surgery and continues to produce beautiful artwork in both his professional life and free time.

Acknowledgements

There are too many individuals who have contributed to this book to mention them all by name. In addition to the authors and editors of this book, there are countless friends, relatives and other individuals who have given up their time to read, comment on and advise about various chapters and sections of the book – to whom we are enormously grateful.

We are grateful to Adam Kanzen who kindly produced the cover illustration and also to Dr Alin Balaj who drew all the illustrations and diagrams within the book. They, like everyone else who helped produce this book, gave their time and expertise for free.

Mel Bezalel undertook the final and extensive proof reading, and members of the forCrohns committee gave invaluable help and advice throughout the process. Through the St Mark's Foundation, whose research forCrohns has supported on several occasions, we were able to secure access to medical professionals with real expertise and interest in Crohn's disease to help write the medical sections. We are grateful to them all.

Finally and most importantly, we would like to thank and acknowledge the enormous courage of the people with Crohn's and their friends and families who took the time to write about their experiences. They did this in the hope that they might help someone they will never meet going through the same difficult time they once did. The moving and personal stories you will read are a generous, selfless act and a testament to their bravery and resilience.

We and they hope that this book will help you.

Section 1

Crohn's disease from the medics

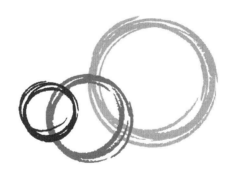

Crohn's disease from the medics

After reading this chapter, we hope you will have a grasp of the basic facts and concepts that will help you to understand Crohn's disease. There is a lot more detail on each area mentioned here in the later chapters, so if something grabs your interest, you can delve a little deeper in section 2 and also get the view from people with Crohn's about that specific issue.

The basics

Crohn's disease is a chronic, inflammatory condition of the bowel. Inflammation means the tissues involved become red, hot, swollen, painful and are unable to do their job well (which, for the bowel means absorbing important nutrients from your food). It is an incurable disease that usually begins in young adulthood and lasts throughout life, with episodes of disease (relapse or flares) and other episodes when the disease is under control (remission).

In Crohn's, the inflammation can occur anywhere in the gut, from the mouth down to the anus, but the most commonly affected areas are the small bowel (ileum) where it joins the large bowel (colon), known as the ileocaecal region, the rest of the colon, the anus and the skin surrounding it (known as the perineum or perianal area).

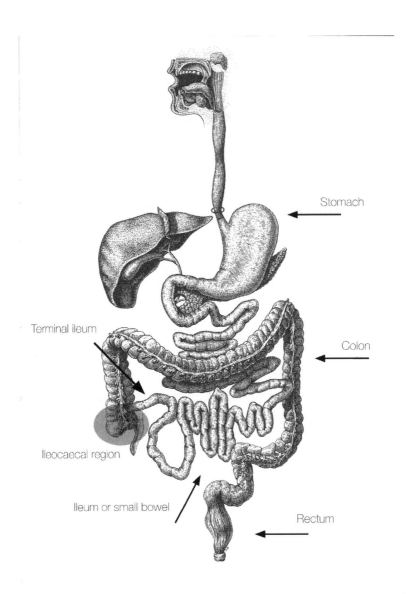

Stomach

Terminal ileum

Colon

Ileocaecal region

Ileum or small bowel

Rectum

Figure 1. The Gastrointestinal tract from mouth to anus. Note the terminal ileum, where the small bowel joins on to the large bowel (colon).

As well as different locations in the gut, Crohn's also affects different people with a different severity of disease. Some people have a relatively mild inflammation, which bothers them from time to time but does not necessarily affect their life much. Others require multiple operations and have problems throughout their lives. The severity of an individual's disease can also change during their lifetime, and reducing severity of symptoms and inducing remission are key goals in the treatment of inflammatory bowel diseases.

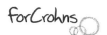

Another form of Inflammatory Bowel Disease (IBD) is Ulcerative Colitis (UC), which affects mostly the colon and does not usually involve the anus or anything other than the last few inches of the small bowel. Irritable Bowel Syndrome (IBS) is totally different and does not involve any inflammation of the bowel, but instead is thought to represent an 'over-excitability' of the bowel – which means that normal stimuli produce disproportionate symptoms such as pain, bloating or a change in bowel habit. It is possible to have both IBS and Crohn's disease.

There are other differences between Crohn's and UC. Some can be seen on special x-ray tests but the most definitive way to tell the difference is through analysis of tissue biopsies under the microscope. However, in spite of these differences, it is sometimes very difficult to tell Crohn's and UC apart.

The precise number of people in the UK suffering with Crohn's disease is not known, although the National Institute of Clinical Excellence suggests it is approximately 115,000. The estimate used by Crohn's and Colitis UK (a national charity for people with IBD) is around 1 in every 650 people, with between 3 and 6000 new cases diagnosed each year.

The disease most commonly first appears during adolescence or early adult life, although it can occur at any point. Men and women are probably equally affected but people of Jewish descent (and particularly Ashkenazi Jews) are disproportionately affected.

It is not known what causes Crohn's disease. There is a genetic component and recent research has identified some genetic abnormalities that make some aspects of Crohn's disease more likely in some people. There is also a higher chance of having Crohn's disease if you have a relative with either Crohn's or UC, but there is no direct inheritance – that means a parent with IBD will not necessarily have a child who is affected, and one child having Crohn's does not mean another child will too. As well as genetic abnormalities, it is generally accepted that people with Crohn's have their normal immune functions disrupted. This might mean that the reaction of a normal person to bacteria in their gut (which is to tolerate the bacteria and allow it to live on the surface of the bowel), is altered in someone with Crohn's – meaning that inflammation occurs in response to normal bacteria, causing damage to the bowel wall itself.

Crohn's disease is not an infection you can catch, nor a condition brought on by bad diet or lifestyle, but there are factors that make some people more likely to have Crohn's than others (like family members with IBD or their ethnicity) and also factors that mean people are more likely to suffer with severe Crohn's (like developing the disease at a younger age or smoking). It is well known that smoking is bad if you have Crohn's disease, increasing the need for surgery, frequency of flares and severity of disease – in fact stopping smoking is one of the single most valuable things a person with Crohn's can do.

Symptoms and diagnosis

The principal symptoms a Crohn's patient may experience include pain in the abdomen (tummy), diarrhoea, sometimes with blood in it and weight loss. A fever may be present, as well as lethargy, and a feeling of being generally unwell or washed out. As you can see, these symptoms are common to many illnesses, including simple gastroenteritis or viral infections and making the diagnosis can be hard. This is discussed more in the Diagnosis chapter. If Crohn's is suspected, doctors are likely to undertake a number of tests to confirm it.

Blood tests may show raised inflammatory markers, which means evidence in the blood of inflammation going on somewhere in the body. Anaemia can occur, and other diseases that can produce similar symptoms (tiredness, diarrhoea, weight loss), such as thyroid problems and coeliac disease (a gluten intolerance disorder), can be ruled out. There is no blood test that can diagnose Crohn's disease. More recently, a test of the patient's stool (poo) has become popular. A protein in the stool called calprotectin can be measured, and if elevated levels are detected, there is a good chance that there is an abnormal process in the bowel causing this. Crohn's disease is only one possible cause of a raised calprotectin level in the stool, but if it is found, doctors will certainly want to undertake further tests such as colonoscopy (discussed below).

Medical imaging tests, using x-rays or scanning techniques, can be very helpful for identifying and 'mapping' the extent of the Crohn's disease. There are several different techniques that you may come across. The old-fashioned but still occasionally useful 'barium' meal and follow through (now more commonly performed with less toxic gastrograffin) uses simple x-rays to examine the bowel – which is outlined on the inside by the gastrograffin (dye that can be seen on x-ray tests). Using this method, thickened, narrowed or ulcerated areas of the bowel can often be seen.

More commonly nowadays, patients will undergo CT or MRI scanning. CT scans also use x-rays, which expose the patient to potentially harmful radiation. However, these scans are often very useful, particularly if the patient comes to hospital having quickly become very unwell. If there is less urgency, then an MRI scan of the bowel can be performed. This uses powerful magnets that shake molecules in your body and detect a signal produced as the molecules return to their original orientation. MRI is excellent for examining soft tissues, and inflammation in the bowel can be effectively assessed.

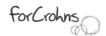

Any imaging, however, shows only a representation of what is happening inside, so the best way to look for inflammation in the lining of the bowel is to look at the lining itself. This is done with a camera test called colonoscopy, in which a long, flexible tube with a camera on the end is passed into the bowel through the anus. It can travel around the colon to the ileocaecal region (where the small and large intestine meet) and it is also possible to take biopsies, small samples of the lining of the bowel, which can then be looked at under the microscope.

The small bowel can also be examined using a camera, although it is not possible to examine the whole small bowel because it is simply too long and too far away from either the mouth or anus, where the tube will be inserted. A small camera contained in a pill (capsule endoscopy) can be swallowed, which takes pictures of the lining of the bowel as it passes through. The pictures are recorded in a pack carried in the pocket and are later analysed back at the hospital.

When investigating for Crohn's disease, any combination of these tests may be used, depending on your symptoms and the location and behaviour of your Crohn's disease. Not all tests are necessary in all patients and your doctor will be able to explain exactly why each is being done.

The behaviour of Crohn's disease

Crohn's disease affects the bowel in discrete segments, with unaffected areas in between patches of inflammation. The inflammation affects the full thickness of the bowel wall, not just the inside lining (mucosa). Ulcerative Colitis, by contrast, tends to affect the bowel in a continuous stretch rather than patches, and affects only the inside lining of the bowel.

After inflammation has occurred, around half of patients with Crohn's move on to a more severe disease form, with what are known as 'stricturing' or 'penetrating' complications. Stricturing means narrowing of the bowel. Since the bowel is a tube through which food and then waste matter passes, narrowings can lead to blockages which we call 'obstruction'. In this situation, patients stop passing so much stool or wind, and the bowel above the blockage swells up rather like when a cartoon character steps on a garden hose. This makes the abdomen swell up and may lead to nausea and/or vomiting.

Penetrating behaviour means that the inflammation leads to a hole in the bowel, which can cause an abscess (a collection of pus) to form next to the hole. This abscess may ultimately find its way out to the skin or another piece of bowel, in which case a tunnel is formed between the two surfaces (bowel and skin, bowel

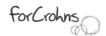

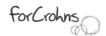

and bowel, bowel and bladder, for example) and this tunnel of infection is called a fistula (which is discussed in the Surgery chapter).

When trying to decide how best to treat someone with Crohn's, it is important to know which part of the bowel is affected and how the disease is behaving. Another particular problem in Crohn's disease is inflammation around the anus, which can also lead to stricturing or formation of an abscess or fistula. These require a slightly different approach to treatment and are all too common. An abscess is a bag of pus, and in this case, it sits next to the anus and swells up to become hot, red and painful. It is usually 'lanced', cut open by a surgeon and allowed to drain, but they sometimes burst on their own. Once opened, the abscess may continue to drain pus, which usually means there is a fistula present, necessitating further surgery or medical treatment.

The increased risk of bowel cancer in some patients with Crohn's disease

In patients with Crohn's disease of the large bowel (colon), called Crohn's Colitis, there can be an increased risk of developing a cancer of the colon. This has long been known in Ulcerative Colitis, but it is now clear that the risk is similar in Crohn's disease. As with UC, the risk is highest with widespread and long-standing Crohn's Colitis, and patients who have the disease limited to the small bowel are not at an increased risk of cancer.

This risk is well understood, and patients who are at risk undergo surveillance colonoscopy to check the colon regularly – in order to look for warning signs that a cancer may be more likely to occur, so that action can be taken early.

Extraintestinal manifestations

As well as the gut, patients with IBD can also have particular problems with the skin, eyes and joints. Perhaps as many as a third (or more) of patients with IBD may have extraintestinal manifestations. Several types of rash are found more commonly in patients with IBD than in other people. Inflammation in the eyes and in the joints (arthritis) also occurs and can be related to a flare of disease in the bowel.

Medical treatment (discussed in more detail in the 'Drugs' chapter)

There are several different types of drugs used in Crohn's disease. They have different roles and are used at different times depending on the severity and behaviour of the disease.

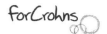

Antibiotics are often used in combination with other drugs and have an effect on symptoms, although it is usually short-lived. 5 ASA drugs such as Mesalazine are anti-inflammatory drugs that can be taken by mouth or as suppositories or enemas direct into the anus if the rectum is inflamed. Azathioprine and 6-Mercapto-purine (6MP) are from the same family of drugs called Thiopurines and are Immunomodulators – which means they suppress the immune system. Some patients cannot tolerate Azathioprine, but find 6-MP effective and tolerable. Steroids have a number of side-effects but can be very quickly effective, particularly in a sudden and severe attack, in which case they may be administered into the vein. Steroid tablets are also effective and are usually stopped in a reducing course over a few days or weeks. Abruptly stopping steroids that have been used for more than a few days is dangerous.

Type of Drug	Examples	Mechanism of action	Side-effects
Antibiotics	Metronidazole	Kill bacteria which might be driving inflammation	Few, mostly mild
Steroids	Prednisolone, Hydrocortisone	Reduce inflammation	Significant, particularly if taken for long periods
Anti-inflammatory drugs	5-ASA, Mesalazine	Reduce inflammation	Mostly mild
Immunosuppressants	Azathioprine, 6MP	Depress the immune system	Some are intolerant of these drugs
Anti TNF agents	Infliximab, Adalimumab	Block TNF alpha activity and reduce inflammation	Unusual but can be severe
Others	Cyclosporin, Methotrexate, Thalidomide	Various	Often very significant side-effects, so these drugs are not often used

Figure 2. Drugs used in Crohn's disease

Other powerful anti-inflammatories or drugs which dampen the immune system (Methotrexate, Cyclosporin, Thalidomide) are used when all else fails. Newer drugs, such as infliximab and adalimumab, which have actually been in regular use for more than a decade, have specific uses in controlling fistulas and maintaining periods of remission. Several of them have significant side-effects which a gastroenterologist would discuss with a patient before they were prescribed, and some of which are discussed in the 'Drugs' chapter.

Diet and nutrition

It is very important for people with Crohn's to have adequate nutrition. Damage to the bowel, inflammation or important sections which have been removed at surgery may mean that someone with Crohn's cannot absorb nutrients through the bowel wall as well as other people – even when in remission. During a flare of the disease, weight can also quickly be lost. Without good nutrition, healing will be slower and the risks of surgery, for example, are increased.

Diet can also be used to treat Crohn's disease. Several types of diet have been produced which in some people have been found to reduce inflammation, often by excluding particular food types or replacing food with carefully designed supplements which provide nutrition but allow the inflammation to settle. Children, in particular, are often treated in this way to prevent exposure to drugs which sometimes have unpleasant side-effects. This is a complex area that is discussed further in the Diet chapter.

Surgery

Surgery cannot be used to cure Crohn's disease. Three quarters of people with Crohn's will need an operation in their lifetime, and some of them will need several operations during their lifetime. It is possible to have so many chunks of bowel removed that in the end, the amount you're left with is not enough to absorb the nutrients from your food properly (which is called intestinal failure due to short bowel syndrome).

Because of this risk, surgeons are very careful when operating on patients with Crohn's disease. The key principles are to remove the diseased segment of bowel but to leave as much healthy bowel as possible in place, and carefully avoid taking any more bowel than is necessary.

Operations are mostly performed when an inflamed segment of bowel has caused a stricture or a fistula. Strictures require removal (if they're long) or widening (if they're short). The narrowed area can be widened by a technique known as stricturoplasty (see Surgery chapter), which avoids removal of any bowel. Fistulas often require removal of the affected segment of bowel and whatever the fistula

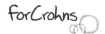

tunnel runs into – which may be another segment of bowel, a patch of skin or a small amount of bladder or vagina.

The most commonly removed area of bowel is the Ileocaecal area, where the large and small bowel meet. This is called right hemicolectomy, although a smaller amount of bowel is usually removed (limited right hemicolectomy or ileocaecal/ileocolic resection). When the chunk of bowel is removed, the two ends of bowel are usually joined together by stitching or stapling the ends. This is called the anastomosis. The main risk following this surgery is that the join can leak, which usually requires a further operation. Unfortunately, this happens slightly more frequently in people with Crohn's than those without, although the risk is usually still low. If the risk of a leak is high, the surgeon may opt to create an ileostomy which is explained below. In order to try and prevent a new flare of Crohn's (which all too often occurs at or just before the site of the join), or at least to delay it, medications such as Azathioprine may be used and further colonoscopy undertaken.

When the large bowel is affected, surgery may also be needed, particularly if there is stricturing or formation of an abscess or fistula. It is also sometimes necessary to remove the problem section of bowel if all attempts to treat it with medication have failed. When a large part of the colon is removed, or if there is significant infection present at the time of operation, or if the patient is very poorly nourished and ill, it is sometimes impossible or unsafe to join the two ends of the bowel back together. In this situation, it is necessary to bring out one end of the bowel onto the skin, like an open mouth which is called a stoma (ileostomy or colostomy). The waste material passes out of the stoma and into a bag stuck to the skin, rather than out through the anus. This can also be used to divert stool away from a section of bowel that has been very inflamed, in the hope that it will improve if there is no stool going past the diseased area every day. Stomas are discussed in more detail in the surgery chapter.

Lifestyle, sex and family

The most important lifestyle factor in Crohn's disease is smoking. Stopping smoking is a good idea for anyone's health, but this is particularly true in the case of Crohn's disease.

Alcohol may lead to a worsening of diarrhoea in some people with Crohn's, just as in some people without IBD, and while excessive alcohol is rarely a good idea, it is safe to drink alcohol in moderation. Alcohol does not cause inflammation or bring about a flare of disease.

Like alcohol, some foods will agree with some people with Crohn's and not with others. There are no fail-safe foods to be eaten by everyone with IBD, nor terrible foods to be avoided by all. If anyone pays attention to their diet, they will notice things that seem to make them feel healthier or more sluggish, or things that seem to make them constipated or have diarrhoea. What you eat does not affect the inflammation in your gut, but as with anyone else, carefully choosing to eat things that seem to agree with you may help with symptoms of diarrhoea and weight loss.

There is no reason for someone with Crohn's disease to avoid exercise. As with anyone else, it is important to avoid dehydration and listen to your body in deciding what exercise to undertake and when, for example, during a flare, it is sensible to take a break.

When it comes to fertility, pregnancy and breast-feeding, there is less evidence about what is safe than we find in other areas which are perhaps easier to study. In general, the advice offered to women by the major gastroenterological associations (like the BSG, British Society of Gastroenterologists) is based on expert opinion rather than proven facts.

Fertility in women with inactive Crohn's disease is similar to other women. Surgery in the pelvis can affect fertility because of scar tissue, which can compress the fallopian tubes (down which the egg passes from the ovary to the womb). Active Crohn's disease can lead to inflammation in the tubes and ovaries as well as around the vagina, which could make conception more difficult. If a woman is in remission when she conceives and is well nourished, this gives her the best chance of staying in remission throughout her pregnancy. A healthy mother is more likely to give birth to a healthy baby, so choosing to get pregnant during a period of remission is sensible. As well as general nutrition, folic acid is important in early pregnancy, and patients with a short bowel or other reasons for not absorbing folic acid well may need a higher dose than other women.

Most women who are in remission at conception will have a normal pregnancy and can give birth via the normal vaginal route. A woman with a stoma can still have a vaginal delivery if they wish. Women who have active inflammation around the anus may want to consider having a Caesarean section to avoid damage to the muscle of the anus, which may already be damaged by Crohn's disease or surgery to the area.

Many of the drugs used in Crohn's disease are probably safe in pregnancy, and many are also probably safe during breast-feeding – this is expanded on further in the Drugs and Having Children chapters. As discussed earlier, there is limited solid evidence because it is not possible (or ethical) to undertake trials

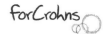

on pregnant women in order to find out which drugs will harm their unborn babies. However, indirect evidence and experience can be used to advise on which drugs are best in pregnancy and breast-feeding. A careful discussion with your gastroenterologist and obstetrician is important so that all the risks can be explained.

Living with Crohn's disease

We hope that this section hasn't frightened you too much! Remember that different people will experience different sets of symptoms and problems, and we have tried to cover a very wide range of the issues in Crohn's disease in a short space. With these basic facts, you can go on and read about drugs, diet, surgery etc. in more detail if or when they apply to you. Most importantly, you can read about the effects they have had on people like you – those with Crohn's and their friends and family, to see how they cope, what helps, what to avoid and how to get through the rough patches. This information, 'straight from the horse's mouth', comes in each chapter after the more detailed medical information and is followed by a few short tips.

Crohn's disease from those with the condition

To share your Crohn's story, please visit forcrohns.org

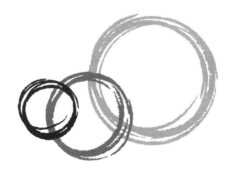

Diagnosis-Hearing those words "you have Crohn's disease"

Being diagnosed with Crohn's disease can create a lot of different feelings: confusion, anxiety and even relief. Crohn's disease is not the easiest condition to diagnose, and the journey to diagnosis itself can take some time. This chapter describes the ways in which it is diagnosed from the point of view of both doctor and patient.

Crohn's disease from the medics

It can be difficult to diagnose Crohn's disease. The symptoms can vary a great deal, from a patient with bloody diarrhoea and pain in their tummy to someone who may have experienced weight loss, a loss of appetite and a feeling of being generally unwell.

As with all medical problems, when trying to decide what is wrong with a patient, a doctor will first take a history of the symptoms, then examine the patient to look for signs of particular diseases and finally undertake 'investigations' (tests). When the results of these are added together, the diagnosis is usually apparent. However, it can be more difficult when there are lots of other diseases with similar symptoms, or when the symptoms are vague and not terribly specific.

Crohn's disease sometimes suffers from both of these problems.

Symptoms and signs

The main symptoms depend on the location of the Crohn's within the bowel, but most commonly, patients will experience diarrhoea (sometimes with blood in), abdominal pain and weight loss. They may also feel generally ill or tired and may have a fever and feel nauseous (sick) or vomit.

The first symptoms can also be those of an acute or severe attack. For example, a patient may come to hospital with pain in the bottom right-hand corner of their tummy – a bit like someone with appendicitis, and may even undergo surgery to remove their appendix, at which point the Crohn's disease is discovered. They may come into hospital with severe pain in their tummy, vomiting and a temperature, perhaps with a lump in their tummy, which their doctor can feel from the outside – due to an abscess (infected collection inside the tummy), or very severe inflammation in the bowel.

On the other hand, the patient may go to their GP with a long history of feeling generally under the weather, tired and mildly unwell. They might have anaemia (lack of red blood cells which makes you feel tired), or weight loss (because they're not absorbing nutrients from their food properly).

There are some features that suggest that an inflammatory bowel disease (Crohn's or Ulcerative Colitis) might be the diagnosis. Having blood relatives with inflammatory bowel disease, having mouth ulcers or having problems around the anus (bottom) such as painful swellings, fissures (little tears) or abscesses (boils, collections of pus) don't mean a patient definitely has Crohn's, but they do make it a more likely diagnosis.

Examination

The doctor will then examine the patient. They will first look at the patient all over, searching for evidence of malnourishment, weight loss, fever or any kind of rash (sometimes associated with inflammatory bowel disease). They will look in the mouth for ulcers and palpate (feel and push gently on) the tummy to look for signs of tenderness (pain on pressing) or for lumps. They will also examine the patient's bottom to look for lumps, fissures and abscesses, and may gently pass a short rigid telescope, called a sigmoidoscope, into the bottom to look for inflammation in the rectum (the last few centimetres of large bowel just above the anus).

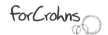

Investigations

Blood tests

First, most doctors will perform blood tests looking for signs of inflammation, anaemia and poor nutrition. They may also look for signs of other diseases, so a wide range of blood tests is often performed at this stage.

Stool tests

Samples of a patient's stool (poo) are often sent to look for evidence of infection, which can cause similar symptoms, especially if there is diarrhoea. A relatively new and increasingly important test at this stage is another stool test, this time looking for a substance called calprotectin (faecal calprotectin). If found in a person's stool, it implies that there may be a disease process in the bowel, and Crohn's is one of the diseases which can lead to a positive test. A positive faecal calprotectin test does not mean a person definitely has Crohn's, but it would make most doctors want to look further with one of the tests discussed below. A negative test makes Crohn's disease less likely (although not impossible).

X-rays

The best tests, and those most likely to make the diagnosis, are those that allow us to look at the bowel and take biopsies (small samples of the bowel). The various imaging tests like X-rays, scans and so on are generally less unpleasant for patients, but do not allow biopsies to be taken. They are sometimes good enough to make a diagnosis of Crohn's disease and are able to look in places that telescopes find it hard to reach, like far up inside the small bowel.

Endoscopic procedures

A colonoscopy (telescope inside the large bowel passed up to reach the end of the small bowel, the terminal ileum) allows doctors to look at the lining of the bowel directly and reveals visible inflammation. It allows doctors to take biopsies that can not only see inflammation that is invisible to the naked eye, but also allows examination of the inflammation under the microscope, which helps doctors tell Crohn's disease apart from other causes of inflammation in the large bowel.

The details: Imaging – x-rays and scans

Crohn's patients may undergo several types of imaging investigation. One small bowel investigation called a barium follow-through is still sometimes useful, but most hospitals would now undertake a scan to examine a patient's bowel. The two most useful types of scan are CT scan and MRI.

CT or computerised tomography scanning uses x-rays fired from the inside of a giant donut. The patient lies on a bed, which moves through the donut with the x-rays being fired every few millimetres of movement, and a computer puts together the information so that a complete image of the patient's body is produced. Drinking lots of water or contrast (dye which shows up on x-rays), and sometimes pumping some air in through the patient's bottom, can help to make the small or large bowel distend (stretch up) a little – making it easier to see what is happening in the bowel itself. The disadvantage is that it uses x-ray radiation, and while having the occasional CT scan is probably low-risk (and is sometimes crucial to keep patients safe), having a lot over a patient's lifetime is thought to increase the risk of getting some types of cancer.

MRI or magnetic resonance imaging does not use x-rays at all. A powerful magnet is used to shake some of the molecules in the body and this movement can be detected by the scanner. Different types of tissue move differing amounts, and a computer can interpret this information and produce an image quite similar to a CT scan. Also like CT, air or water can be used to improve the picture of the bowel obtained – this is sometimes called MR enterography or enteroclysis.

MRI is better at looking for some problems than CT and vice versa. In an emergency situation, a CT is faster and often more useful, but when speed or urgency are not so important, an MRI scan is often a better test. Your doctor will be able to explain why they are choosing one particular type of scan over another. Some people find MRI scanners claustrophobic and noisy. People who have some types of metal in their eyes or bodies cannot have MRI scans because the magnet may move this metal and cause damage.

Endoscopy

Endoscopy is the use of a camera to examine parts of the body from the inside. The most common endoscopic procedure in Crohn's is colonoscopy, although it is also possible to examine the stomach with a gastroscope, or the small bowel with advanced endoscopy techniques either using a long colonoscope or a camera contained in a pill. A patient can swallow this, and it transmits pictures taken every few seconds to a box carried in their pocket, which their doctor can download and examine afterwards.

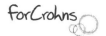

Colonoscopy

Before colonoscopy, patients have to drink 'prep' – a strong laxative to empty the bowel completely so that the lining of the bowel can be examined. It causes diarrhoea, which empties the bowel in the 24 hours prior to the test.

The colonoscope is a long, thin black telescope with a fibre optic camera on the end. It can be passed in through the anus and around the large bowel right up to the end of the small bowel (terminal ileum). Pain-killers and sedative drugs are often used to make the procedure more comfortable. As well as looking at the bowel, a doctor can take pictures, videos and also small biopsies – samples of the tissue taken with little forceps (like a tiny mouth that takes a small bite of the tissue of the bowel), which can be collected and examined under the microscope.

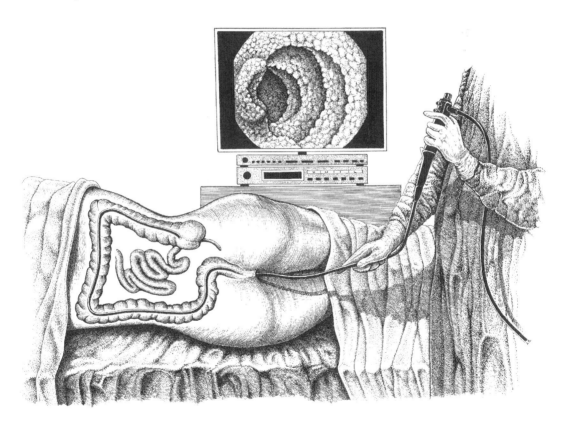

Figure 3. Colonoscopy

The biopsies are examined (this is called histology) to look for features typical of Crohn's disease. Other diseases such as Ulcerative Colitis, some infections of the bowel and other rarer diseases can also be identified by histology.

The diagnosis

At the end of this process, a diagnosis of Crohn's can often be made, but sometimes the features are unclear and despite a doctor suspecting Crohn's, they may not have enough evidence to be sure. If Crohn's is diagnosed, treatment can be started and this will depend on the location of the Crohn's disease and the form it takes (behaviour). For example, a stricture (narrowing) at the end of the small bowel, where it joins the large bowel (terminal ileum), would be treated differently to inflammation in the middle of the small bowel with no narrowing.

Crohn's disease can change location and behaviour. For this reason, these tests are often repeated during a patient's lifetime, particularly if symptoms change, so that treatment can also be modified if necessary. This process is called mapping the extent of the disease and allows us to classify a patient's disease.

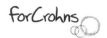

Crohn's disease from the patients

The following section looks at the experiences of five people when they were diagnosed with Crohn's. For all of them, the diagnosis comes after suffering from the symptoms for some time and this is often the case, although increasingly, the path to diagnosis should become smoother and quicker. The various tests and initial treatments are also discussed and it's worth remembering that not all of these are relevant for any given individual – some are necessary for some people and others not.

Claire

Claire is 23 and a nursing student. She is single and was diagnosed with Crohn's eight years ago

"I started losing weight about six months before I was diagnosed, but I put it down to having to walk an hour to school every day. Looking back however, I probably had mild symptoms as young as eight, but my parents just didn't think anything of it as I was always a sickly child.

My mum started getting concerned with *the weight loss* [1] and we had many arguments about it because she was convinced I had anorexia. Eventually I went to the doctor, who completely fobbed me off; they didn't seem concerned that I was only five stone at 15. I didn't even have a blood test and was instantly told I had *irritable bowel syndrome* [2], was given *Buscopan* [3] and sent away.

Time went by with no improvement and I was forced to wear clothes for nine-year-old girls. At this point, I wasn't experiencing any toilet

1. Phil (Gastro) says:
Although unexplained or unintended weight loss can be caused by many things, it is an important barometer of disease activity in people with Crohn's disease. In people with diarrhoea, and other gastrointestinal symptoms, if accompanied by weight loss, your GP should refer you to a specialist immediately.

2. Phil (Surgeon) says:
Irritable Bowel Syndrome (IBS) is completely different to Inflammatory Bowel Diseases (IBD, including Crohn's disease and Ulcerative Colitis) although some symptoms are similar. In IBS, there is no inflammation or change to the structure of the bowel so a colonoscopy or scan can often tell the difference between the two.

3. Phil (Surgeon) says:
Buscopan is an antispasmodic drug used to calm the bowel and relieve cramps. It can be used in both IBS and IBD.

symptoms, just weight loss. I eventually got to see a lady doctor who was very concerned and thought I was depressed. She agreed to refer me to Birmingham children's hospital. I met a gastroenterologist, who said he only had to look at me to diagnose Crohn's disease.

At this point, I was 15 and oblivious. I had never heard of the disease and assumed it was nothing serious. I don't think I even did any research to find out what it was. I found at that age that I just did as I was told and took the tablets I was supposed to, without asking questions. I had nobody to talk to who knew about the disease. I don't think I even talked about it until I was 18, as *I felt very embarrassed* [4] and people didn't want to take the time to learn about it, so I thought there was no point in trying. It wasn't until I started my nursing training that I took the time to find out about my disease. I only really started talking about it a year ago, when I joined Twitter and finally found people who had the same disease and understood how I felt. It felt like a weight had been lifted. I would have loved to have had the support back when I was 15, which is why I am so keen to help young people with IBD, as I think they should get more support."

> **4. Lucy (IBD Nurse) says:**
> Patients can often feel embarrassed and alone when first diagnosed, but the IBD nurses and doctors are there to support patients through this, and help put them in touch with other patients or support groups.

Deepan

Deepan is 23. He is currently studying childcare. Here he tells the story of his diagnosis.

"I've suffered from Crohn's disease for about 12 years. It all began in June of 2000. I remember the afternoon like it was yesterday. I was wrestling with my cousins in the garden before a family BBQ and I must have fallen to the ground under a pile-up. I got up, brushed myself off, proceeded to land some punches on everyone within reach and thought nothing more of it. The next few days were OK, maybe my appetite wasn't up to scratch but I'd just put that down to the good weather and wanting to be outside playing (yes outside, not inside playing video games! Oh Em Gee).

Then the weekend came... and every other day for the next six months. I was doubled up in pain, in the foetal position, driving to and from various A&E

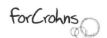

departments across west London. I ended up seeing junior doctors either at the beginning, middle or end of their 24/36 hour shifts. Despite my best efforts to explain in graphic detail why I was there, and what I was feeling like to get me in that position, they had no real idea of what they were doing. All that came were endless blood tests and painkillers. I was once even told in true school P.E. teacher fashion to "walk it off"! Eventually my parents and *I lost hope in the NHS's competency in diagnosing the ailment and we contacted a private healthcare provider* [5] that my father's ex-employer had set up for him way back when.

We (my dad and I) dutifully went to the first appointment at a prestigious West London Hospital. Up to the 5th Floor. Very plush and pompous. I sat down and explained my symptoms: pain, nausea, weight loss, lethargy, diarrhoea, blood in the stools etc. Without saying anything, *he ordered a specific blood test (of which I was now accustomed to) and a stool (poo) test* [6]. We were asked, very politely, to go and get a hot drink and something to eat for an hour or two, while the results came in. We were sat in the hospital restaurant having a cup of tea and waiting for the verdict or diagnosis of some kind when, true to his word, a phone call came on my dad's mobile asking us to come back up.

Once sat down, we were given the diagnosis: Crohn's disease. What I would've given for any kind of smart phone at that moment! Being told felt weird. He said that it wasn't something that would normally kill you but couldn't be fixed by a course of antibiotics. I didn't know what to feel. Surprised, curious, angry? Mostly I felt relieved to know that the problem had a name, but also scared out of my mind because I didn't know what Crohn's disease actually was. The leaflets were of

5. Phil (Gastro):
Whilst it is sad to hear Deepan's story and his initial impression of his treatment in the NHS, the vast majority of Crohn's patients are treated in the NHS. In fact, it is more than likely his consultant in the private sector works within the NHS and looks after many Crohn's patients in the NHS. The most important thing was that Deepan got to see a Gastroenterologist – whether that was in the NHS or a private hospital.

6. Phil (Surgeon) says:
This blood test would not definitively tell the doctor that Deepan had Crohn's but it would have been another piece of the jigsaw added to Deepan's history and the things the doctor found when he examined him. The only definite way to diagnose Crohn's is by taking a biopsy (looking at a piece of the bowel under the microscope) but there is often enough information from history, blood tests and scans to make the diagnosis clear without a biopsy.

little help because my mind was still processing the conversation we had just had. Who, what, when, where, why, how?

The drive home was quiet. I didn't know what to say. It felt like a kick in the teeth because we knew what it was, but at the same time we didn't. We stopped off at a local library when we got close to home, just to see if we could find some, if *any information about Crohn's.* [7] We didn't. No huge surprise there.

When we got home, my dad read my mind and fired up the computer and the slow dial-up connection, which at this point, I felt like throwing out of the window. I thought that if I walked to the central library, got a book on Crohn's and walked back with a cup of tea from McDonalds, I'd get home before the computer managed to find something. Thankfully I decided to avoid that course of action, and sat patiently waiting for the search page to load up. This seemed like the longest 10 minutes of my life. The familiar sound of the modem dialling the number to access the internet began to sound like a rhythmic tune in my head and I was beginning to drown out all outside noises and people. I must have been day-dreaming when my dad put his hand on my shoulder telling me to start typing.

C- r –o- h- n ' s d- i- s- e- a -s - e I read the spelling out loud to make sure there weren't any mistakes. Inflammatory Bowel Disease. Ulcers. *Can be severe. Intestinal Failure. Stoma* [8]. These were some of the phrases and words that began to pop up on pages all over the place.

7. Phil (Surgeon) says:
Seeking information is a valuable thing, but it's important to be able to understand what the information means. Crohn's disease can be mild or severe, it can affect different parts of the bowel; some people need surgery, others don't. Remember that when reading about Crohn's, you are reading about someone else's experience, not necessarily the experience you will have.

8. Phil (Gastro) says:
The words that Deepan describes are all extremely emotive as they describe the most severe end of the Crohn's disease 'spectrum' which can be very frightening before more information and knowledge is known about the individual condition. Deepan will most likely have had a colonoscopy procedure and other x-ray investigations to establish the extent of his individual disease, just as almost all patients who are just diagnosed with Crohn's disease do.

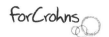

The one phrase that stood out for me was *"intestinal failure"* [9] - what did that mean? Would they remove my intestine? How would I digest food? More importantly, how would I dispose of it? I'd already lost so much weight, I didn't fancy losing any more.

The next few days, things got better, as I understood more about what Crohn's was, but they were also daunting as I began to come to terms with the fact that there is no cure. Yet..."

Patrick

Patrick is 37, married with one child and works as a software developer. He was diagnosed at the age of 16, and after a period of severe Crohn's, is currently in remission.

> **9. Phil (Surgeon) says:**
> Intestinal failure is a condition in which your bowel is not able to absorb adequate nutrients or water to sustain healthy life. It occurs when a lot of bowel has been removed or has become diseased, and it is a well-known but uncommon problem in Crohn's disease. Surgeons are careful to avoid removing too much bowel and medical treatments are geared at trying to preserve the bowel. With intestinal failure, supplementary nutrition is provided into the vein (discussed in more detail in the Drugs chapter).

"For as long as I can remember, I've had abdominal pain. And for even longer, I've thought that this was normal. I had no reason to believe that I was sick or otherwise, but this was a daily occurrence. By the age of 13, my symptoms had grown to include *diarrhoea, extreme tiredness, nausea and increasing pain* [10] in the morning and complete loss of appetite. My bowels became more and more urgent, and I sometimes felt that I wouldn't make it to the bathroom in time. I had no idea what was going on. At the time I didn't talk to my parents about it, I just tried to deal with it on my own. My pain became so intense that I couldn't get up in the morning. I missed several days of

> **10. Phil (Surgeon) says:**
> These are classic symptoms of Crohn's disease, although they could represent other diseases too. Part of the trouble is that symptoms like pain, nausea, loss of appetite and weight are very non-specific.

school, my grades plummeted, my growth was slowed and I lost a lot of weight. At 13, I weighed about 90 pounds. My parents started to get concerned and asked questions. I told them about my symptoms and they asked me why I hadn't come to them sooner. The symptoms were so gradual that I really didn't think it was out of the ordinary. I know that sounds absurd, but at that age I just tried to be normal and it never occurred to me that I was seriously ill.

We went to my family physician who referred us to a gastroenterologist. Within days of the consultation, I was scheduled for *a colonoscopy*. [11] The preparation for this test was horrible and painful. The salty liquid was like drinking sea water but that wasn't as bad as what followed. Within a few hours, I had more abdominal pain and I was quick to rush to the bathroom where Niagara Falls cleared out my system.

The actual colonoscopy wasn't too bad. For the first time in my life, I had anaesthetic, which was a *weird floating-on-a-cloud feeling*. [12] I didn't feel a thing. Shortly thereafter, my gastroenterologist met my parents and me, and gave us the conclusion to the test. I had Crohn's disease."

Ruth

Ruth is 55 years old and was diagnosed with Crohn's disease 30 years ago. She is now a part-time bookkeeper and has two children, 26 and 22. Here she tells the story of her diagnosis.

"My story starts in 1982 when I was 25, and married for just a year. I had suffered numerous stomach pains throughout my teenage years but was told by my parent's doctor that I had Monday morning tummy – worried about school!

11. Phil (Surgeon) says:
A colonoscopy is a camera or telescope test. A long, flexible tube is passed in through the anus and up and round the bowel, all the way to the terminal ileum (where the small and large bowel meet). Any inflammation in the bowel can be examined and biopsies (tiny pieces of bowel wall to be examined under the microscope) taken.

12. Phil (Gastro) says:
During a colonoscopy most people are given sedation via a 'drip' (cannula) in their arm. The sedation is to help relax the patient but is not a general anaesthetic whereby the person is not conscious during the procedure. Patients can be given a pain killer as well as they can sometimes feel bloated from the air that is used to expand the bowel during the procedure.

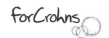
forCrohns

I suffered an abscess in my rectum in October 1980, and after a very painful operation to remove it, there was no mention that this could have been *a cause of Crohn's*. [13] My sister had been diagnosed with Crohn's some years earlier, so I was told to see the consultant who had diagnosed hers.

After seeing him, he said I did not need any tests as it wasn't Crohn's, but I had an aortogram which showed I had a *narrowed artery leading to the bowel* [14] – which needed to be inflated so the blood could flow properly. A date was set for this operation. My late father was talking to a cousin in the States who specialises in blood, and he told my dad that it could not be this as the pain I described would not be this bad. We insisted on seeing the surgeon again and told him. At this point he then said it probably wasn't this and the pains were in my head and I should see a psychiatrist. We left immediately as that was what my sister went through years earlier!

The pain continued on and off, and by around December 1982, the pain was unbearable. I had been so ill over the Christmas period that I'd cancelled all plans, but my ex-husband and I were due to go to a fancy dress party on New Year's Eve and I insisted on going. As I was getting ready, I felt a sharp pain that took my breath away because of its intensity and made me stop in my tracks. My ex rang the hospital, and they said I should take peppermint tablets as it was probably indigestion. After a few minutes, the pain went, and although I felt like death warmed up, we went to the party.

A few days later, I was sick and incontinent. I was rushed to hospital and later that night was operated on for peritonitis, and given a blood transfusion. Not only had my *appendix* [15] erupted, but it was

13. Phil (Surgeon) says:
The abscess will not have caused the Crohn's but abscesses around the anus and rectum are very common in Crohn's disease (see surgery chapter). It was certainly sensible, given this and Ruth's family history, to seek advice.

14. Phil (Surgeon) says:
This is called mesenteric ischaemia. It is not associated with Crohn's disease.

15. Phil (Surgeon) says:
The appendix is a small, worm-like bit of bowel that sticks off the large bowel where the small bowel joins it. It is common to get appendicitis, and this is not related to Crohn's disease, although the symptoms can be similar. If it bursts or goes gangrenous, peritonitis can occur which is inflammation of the whole of the inside of the abdomen – this is a very serious problem requiring immediate surgery.

gangrenous. I also needed an iron infusion, which didn't agree with me. By this stage, I weighed only five and a half stone. As I left hospital a few days later, my family commented that I looked like someone needing admission, not discharge. I was back in shortly afterwards, for a *pelvic abscess* [16], which luckily dispersed by itself.

The pain continued, along with rushing to the loo many, many times a day. My late dad had had enough, and insisted I see a private doctor. Early in 1983, I was admitted to a London hospital and had two weeks of tests, including a *barium meal and follow through, IVP, ultra sound scan and barium meal enema* [17] before being told I had Crohn's disease. I was told that because it was so bad, it was too late to be treated with medication and I would have to be operated on. Although it was devastating news, it actually came as a relief to be told what it was. The diagnosis *was "Crohn's disease of the terminal ileum and proximal colon"* [18].

I was in for a further two weeks (four weeks in all), 3ft of intestine – some small and large – was taken away. After coming out of hospital three days later, I was admitted again with terrible pain. My surgeon had to leave a dinner party to operate on an abscess that was under the scar tissue. A further three and a half weeks in hospital.

16. Phil (Surgeon) says:
This is quite common after peritonitis and often does resolve, particularly if small. Sometimes antibiotics or drainage under guidance of a scan is required.

17. Phil (Surgeon) says:
These tests are discussed in more detail earlier in the chapter. The barium meal and follow through and barium enema involve putting barium up the bum or getting the patient to swallow it. X-rays are taken and the barium coats the wall of the bowel – if there are ulcers or lumps on the lining of the bowel, or particularly narrowings or fistulas, these can be seen. These findings in the small bowel are typical of Crohn's disease.

18. Phil (Surgeon) says:
This is the classic location for Crohn's to affect, and the operation to remove the end of the ileum and start of the colon is called a right hemicolectomy. The minimum amount of bowel is removed. More details can be found in chapter 3.

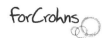

Since then, I have been in pretty good health with just a few hiccups. The worst outcome of my operations has been the *constant need for the loo*" [19a+b].

Karen

Karen is 31 and is a contract engineer. She was diagnosed with Crohn's at 24 and describes her condition as 'mild'. She has not had any operations for her Crohn's. Here she describes the lead up to her diagnosis:

"I didn't really see it coming. To be honest, I don't think I knew what Crohn's disease was until my diagnosis in 2005. How did it come about? I began to notice myself losing weight. I hadn't been watching what I was eating and certainly wasn't exercising excessively either. Was I stressed? I guess I always was a worrier and stressed from time to time, but that's just my nature. I started noticing my toilet trips were increasing, particularly after meals. I realised I wasn't getting any energy from the food I was digesting, as 30 minutes after a meal, there it was in the toilet. (Sorry if that's too much information but its true).

I thought "Hmm, maybe I've eaten too much Bran Flakes today? Or maybe I'm stressed about something? Maybe it's just a large bout of diarrhoea or a stomach bug passing?" I thought, 'I'm going to watch what I eat', so I started to cut right back on foods containing a lot of fibre and avoided spicy foods. I started on white bread and pasta for dinner but yet again, off I went to the toilet half an hour later. Don't get me wrong, the weight loss was fab for a while! I thought: "great, I can eat anything I want, even chocolate and don't gain any weight from it, woo hoo!"

19a. Phil (Surgeon) says:
This can occur following right hemicolectomy, but can also be part of the Crohn's disease itself.

19b. Phil (Gastro) says:
Post operatively it is likely the majority of Ruth's care will be under the gastroenterology team (medical team) and the cause of her urgency to go to the toilet will be investigated typically to see if her Crohn's disease has returned, or whether there is another cause for her symptoms such as not absorbing her bile salts (which can sometimes happen after the end of the small bowel (ileum) is removed). This can be treated by simple medications to reduce the urgency

How stupid of me to think that! I noticed the weight falling off rapidly, but I also noticed I was suffering from a hell of a lot of *mouth ulcers* [20]! Even Bonjela failed to get rid of these nasties appearing each day. I remember having 4-5 ulcers in my mouth at a time. I finally went to the doctor, as I became very worried about these symptoms. I felt drained and was getting no energy from food. Within a week, I was at the hospital receiving a colonoscopy to find out what was going on in there. An hour later, I was sat with my consultant, being told I was suffering from Crohn's disease. They had discovered a lot of ulcers present on my bowel. I was told my condition was quite serious and was immediately put on a course of steroids.

How did I feel when I was given my diagnosis? Confused to start with; I couldn't figure out why I had been diagnosed with the illness. As far as I was aware, no one in my family had been diagnosed with it. I didn't really know what Crohn's disease was. I thought I was just stressed out and my stomach had gone into overdrive mode with nervous butterflies, but this wasn't the case. My Dad went out and bought me an informative book on the illness, which contained stories of other sufferers. I guess it was a way of helping me digest the illness and show me I was not alone in my suffering[21]. I didn't know anyone else who had this condition to ask them about it. *It felt a bit lonely to be honest.*

The depression then kicked in[22]; it went on for months afterwards. Nothing that required anti-depressants, but I felt very down about myself. My self-confidence dipped and I wondered 'Why me?' I wondered if the illness had been lying dormant in my body, waiting to surprise me one day? It felt like it...

20. Phil (Surgeon) says:
Mouth ulcers can appear in people without Crohn's, but the disease can cause ulceration in the mouth and recurrent or numerous ulcers may be a sign of Crohn's disease.

21. Lucy (IBD Nurse) says:
When people have first received a diagnosis of Crohn's disease, the gastroenterologist, surgeon or IBD nurse can provide additional information from charities such as forCrohns to help explain the disease and its treatment.

22. Phil (Gastro) says:
Depression and stress is common in patients with Crohn's disease, especially if the disease is very active and severe. Patients should inform their gastroenterology doctors, IBD nurse or GP if they feel low, depressed or stressed as additional support can be given. This is covered in detail in the Psychology chapter.

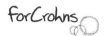

Before my diagnosis, I was a very sociable person and liked to keep fit at the gym regularly, always on the go. After my diagnosis, I soon realised that I couldn't do everything all the time, or take on too much. I was off work for a few weeks initially, and then reduced my work hours; but I went back full-time after the steroids helped me recover.

The hardest part for me was accepting I had a chronic condition and the uncertainty surrounding it, with flare-ups and treatments, as there is no cure. It got me down a lot, as the hardest part for me was the tiredness and fatigue I used to suffer from.

Looking back, I've learnt that the key is to try to remain positive, never take anything for granted and make the most of life. If anything, having this condition has made me want to push myself more and do all the things I wanted to do. Never think you have to deal with this condition alone."

Summary

Diagnosing Crohn's disease can be difficult and may take some time because the symptoms are often vague and not very specific. It is often when a gastroenterologist or colorectal surgeon is involved that the right investigations are performed, which lead to the answer – and this is done in the NHS as well as private hospitals. The tests can be unpleasant, but they all have a purpose, and your doctor can explain exactly what they hope to see when a test is recommended. 'Mapping' the extent of your disease helps your doctor to recommend the right treatment and may need to be done several times through your life as your symptoms change.

Tips and suggestions

The following tips and suggestions are taken from our healthcare professionals and those with Crohn's disease.

- **If you think it could be Crohn's, say so**
  If you're worried that you may have Crohn's disease when visiting the doctor with symptoms, say so.

- **Mention all of your symptoms**
  Always mention all your symptoms. Subtle symptoms may have been troubling you for some time, even if your diarrhoea, for example, is quite new. Try and recall the last time you were completely well and record any symptoms.

- **If you are having any tests understand what they are and why you're having them**
  When your doctor organises a test, ask about the associated risks and what it will show you. They will be able to give a good explanation of why you're having it and how it will help which may make it easier to tolerate if it is unpleasant.

- **Follow-up if you've been waiting too long for test results**
  You should expect to hear from the relevant department (Radiology or Endoscopy) within a few weeks of your test being requested – if you haven't heard, call your consultant's secretary who can check with them that all is well and pre-empt any problems.

- **Colonoscopy Tests**
  The prep for a colonoscopy will give you diarrhoea. Follow the instructions given by the endoscopy department carefully and be sure to drink enough water as you can get dehydrated if you don't. You'll need someone to pick you up after the test as you can't drive after having the sedative drugs and may not feel like walking or getting the bus.

- **Keep a diary of your symptoms**
  If finding the diagnosis is proving difficult, keep a diary of your symptoms to show the doctor next time you see them. This might mean you can demonstrate a pattern of symptoms that helps guide the doctor towards the correct diagnosis.

- **Seek out advice and information**
  At the back of this book, in section 5, there are links and contact details to further sources of information and useful organisations.

Everyday life

Crohn's disease affects people in different ways on a day to day basis and individuals find their own tips and strategies to help them manage their condition each day. This chapter looks at a range of stories to explain how Crohn's can impact on routines and habits, or elements of everyday living such as going on holiday and shows the different ways those with Crohn's seek to stay in control of their condition, where possible.

Crohn's disease from the medics

The impact of Crohn's disease on everyday life is determined by the symptoms a patient has at any given time. During periods of remission, there may be few or no symptoms at all. During relapse, however, the symptoms encountered can certainly have an impact.

The principle symptoms which might influence the life of someone with Crohn's include frequent and loose bowel motions, difficulty in controlling these motions, abdominal (tummy) pain, weakness, tiredness, nausea and loss of weight.

Inflammation in the bowel produces a runny, liquid stool (bowel motion) - diarrhoea. This can mean that some people will open their bowels many times a day and, during a bad flare of disease, perhaps 20 or more times. Even a normal day might mean several trips to the loo to pass a loose stool. This can lead to embarrassment and inconvenience, especially during meetings, commuting or in open offices. A liquid stool is more difficult to control, especially if the lower rectum or anus is inflamed, and as a result many people feel 'urgency' – the need to get to the loo as soon as they have the urge to go, with very little warning at all.

Pain in the tummy is caused by inflammation, or sometimes by spasm if the bowel is 'held up' or partially obstructed by a narrowed area (stricture), and can range from mildly annoying to debilitating.

Specific problems can be caused by anal Crohn's disease, which can make sitting and walking uncomfortable or embarrassing. Stomas can be noisy and occasionally they can leak or smell. Medical treatments and surgery may also have a significant impact on life at the time and afterwards; the influence of these is discussed in the Drugs and Surgery chapters.

Surgical wounds may heal slowly in Crohn's disease, and a partially unhealed wound may have implications for activities such as swimming, exercise and particular kinds of work. Inflammation in the joints (arthritis) or skin, associated with Crohn's disease and present in some sufferers, can lead to difficulty with physical activity of any sort.

When someone with Crohn's is having a flare-up of the disease (when the inflammation becomes more severe), there can be several specific effects. As well as often having diarrhoea, they tend to eat less, which means they absorb fewer nutrients and may become dehydrated. This leads to feelings of weakness, tiredness and often loss of weight. They may also find that some foods make their symptoms worse or struggle with their diet, trying to decide what's good and bad for them.

We have probably all felt something like this for a day or two from time to time, when we get 'food poisoning' or gastroenteritis. However, Crohn's disease can cause prolonged episodes of (sometimes severe) symptoms which patients battle through and live with in order to maintain everyday life.

Crohn's disease from the patients

These stories reflect the impact Crohn's has on the day-to-day life of several people who suffer from Crohn's – in particular looking at their working lives, commuting and day-to-day activities.

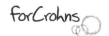

Paul

Paul is 36, married with two young kids and was diagnosed with Crohn's disease in 2006. His Crohn's started with a never-ending stomach ache on his honeymoon. After two courses of antibiotics and four months of pain, he was finally diagnosed, but didn't respond to any of the medication and needed emergency surgery to remove 10 inches of his small bowel that year.

"Whilst I'm relatively pain-free these days, Crohn's is with me 24/7, 365 days a year. Ever since my initial surgery, I've suffered with diarrhoea, particularly in the mornings. The doctor said that it can take the bowel 12 months to adjust to having a shorter bowel; well I'm still waiting! I live on the outskirts of London, but my office is in central London and I regularly make 100 mile trips down the motorway to my other office. It's these every day commutes that everyone else takes for granted that I can't. It's rare that I can leave the house before 8.30 in the morning; my bowels just won't allow it. And even then, once I've walked the eight minutes to my nearest tube station, my first stop is the toilet there. Fortunately, the line I take is well-prepared, with toilets at pretty much every station, and I know exactly where they are if I need one. Transport for London produces a map that shows which stations have them, and there's a handy iPhone app called 'Loo Tube' for when I'm veering off my usual path. It's probably the best 69p I've ever spent! All the toilets have different challenges. Some are free, some need a 20p piece and others a 50p (I keep a healthy supply of change in my pocket so you can probably hear me jangling on the Jubilee Line), some take Radar keys, and then of course there's the usual mix of well-maintained and filthy toilets. But beggars can't be choosers. I would say that 90 per cent of my morning tube journeys involve a trip to the loo. I build that time into my work schedule, so it's rare for me to book a meeting before 10am, for fear of being late. I'm very open about my condition with my colleagues, so they know if I'm late, or need to duck out of a meeting, it's probably down to my guts. Fortunately, my current boss knows a fair bit about the condition, so that has made things easier for me, too.

My biggest worry is that I get stuck somewhere, and if the train does stop, that's when the psychological challenges come into play. I automatically go into panic mode and feel I need the loo even when I probably don't. I try and force myself to stay on the train once we start moving, but the fear of being caught short inevitably ends up with me getting off to find the loo – just to be safe. Incidentally, some of the loos on the tube are before the barriers and I've found that staff are really helpful if you explain your situation - it certainly saves a few quid on my Oyster card!

When I'm driving on the motorway, the fear of a jam and getting stuck is always there. To get round this, I try and leave by 6.30am at the latest, but my bowels can be unreliable – even when I wake up at five! I always check the traffic reports before I leave, and stay tuned to the radio, while my satnav shows all the petrol and service stations in case of emergencies.

I have to fly to meetings in Europe quite regularly too. Early morning flights are the norm, and again, that's always a worry until I reach the safety of the airport. Sometimes I'll take an Imodium tablet, as the fear starts again at take off when the seat belt signs go on, but it's mainly psychological and I don't actually need to go. Being abroad presents its own challenges, of course. Explaining to taxi drivers that I need them to stop for me means I always go prepared with the relevant local translations, but toilets aren't as well located in most other countries and they certainly aren't as clean! On a recent trip to Poland, I was suddenly desperate for the loo. I hadn't done my homework so didn't know the Polish word for 'toilet'.

By the time I'd figured that out and found the loo, I discovered I needed a one zloty coin to open the door! Cue panic, which only exacerbated the feeling in my guts, but as always, I eventually got myself sorted and didn't get caught out. I learnt my lesson, that's for sure – always be prepared.

You may be thinking "why doesn't he eat less before he flies or not eat risky foods", but the trouble is I've never managed to figure out what foods cause me trouble. I can have a curry one day and be fine the next, and then a sandwich the next night and be stuck the following morning. There's just no pattern and it's the unpredictability that causes the unnecessary worrying. I'm lucky that once it gets to lunchtime I'm usually fine for the rest of the day. That's why I try and plan all my meetings and particularly big presentations for the afternoon. I've never been a morning person and the Crohn's has certainly not helped that.

Outside of work, I try to live my life as normally as I possibly can, *and don't let Crohn's get in the way if there's something I want to do* [1]. Whilst I'm a bit

1. Phil (Gastro) says:
Paul's story is very common as many people with Crohn's disease persevere with their daily activities by being vigilant and knowing where the nearest toilets are. The urge to go to the toilet, and the triggers for this can range from active disease, to irritable bowel syndrome (IBS) which can co-exist in patients with Crohn's, through to malabsorption of bile salts. It is important for your gastroenterologist to know about these symptoms as there may be treatments to help reduce the distressing and annoying sudden urge to dash to the toilet.

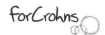

older now and I'm not out clubbing or going to gigs every week, if there's an event I want to go, to I will try and go. I go to football regularly, and as you'd expect, there aren't enough toilets for everyone in the stadium – so there are often long queues. There's a disabled toilet that is manned by a steward, so only those in wheelchairs can access it, but I've spoken to the club's customer services manager and they gladly provided me with a letter which means I can use that toilet if I have to.

My mates all know about my condition and it's a regular topic of conversation; I'm often the butt (no pun intended) of jokes. I think they are all a bit jealous of my Radar key to be honest!

In the seven years I've had this rotten disease, I've not been caught short once... yet. And whilst I'm not a fan of those posters that say "Keep Calm, It's Only..." if there's any advice I could offer to another sufferer in situations like those I've outlined above it would be to try and stay calm and think to yourself "Keep Calm, It's Only Crohn's disease".

Claire

Claire is 27 and was first diagnosed with Crohn's at the age of nine. She currently works as a private nanny. Here she explains some of the problems Crohn's has brought to her day-to-day life, as well as her coping mechanisms.

"At first, it was hard to explain to people what Crohn's was, but once I became familiar with it, I never had a problem admitting that I had this disease.

School trips were tricky and I refused to stay at my friends' houses overnight, due to fear of needing the toilet urgently. To this day, I still suffer with big anxiety attacks when I am out of my comfort zone. I struggle to leave my local area and I have had to fly home early from a holiday before, due to this anxiety. It's not fun, but with help, I'm slowly learning to deal with it.

My job is local because I couldn't think of anything worse than travelling on public transport on a daily basis. What do I do if we get stuck? What do I do if I need the toilet urgently? I avoided underground trains for the first 15 years after my diagnosis. My fear was huge and there was no way anyone, or anything, would get me on London Underground. But earlier this year, I finally conquered my fear and travelled to central London by tube. It wasn't as bad as I had thought (this seems to happen with a lot of 'new' things I try), but then again, I didn't need the toilet in that short space of time.

I also hadn't been to a concert in an arena, or stadium, or a theatre show since I was diagnosed. And again, earlier this year I did it. I was bought a ticket for a concert at Wembley Stadium, along with 80,000 other people. The tickets were paid for, so how could I say no? When we arrived at the stadium (or anywhere I go that's unfamiliar), the first thing I had to do was familiarise myself with the nearest toilet. I have a Radar key which unlocks many disabled toilets, so this helps me a lot when in busy, public places and I just don't have 'time' to queue.

I'm recently engaged and my fiancé has been very supportive of my illness. When I first told him about it (probably on our first date!), it was a bit daunting, but he later told me that he went home that evening and researched it online to understand a bit more. He realised it wasn't a 'serious' condition, but I did have to explain that it debilitates each person differently, and although I haven't had any surgery, it still affects me every day. My biggest daily symptom is that when I have to go to the toilet, I HAVE to go to the toilet! I count myself lucky that this is usually as bad as it gets on a day-to-day basis. Living with Crohn's isn't so bad. As long as you know how to control it as best as you can, and surround yourself with loving, caring and understanding people, you can live life to the full – exactly like everyone around you!"

Kath

Kath was diagnosed with Crohn's in August 2010 and underwent surgery a few months later. Here she reflects on the impact of Crohn's on her life.

"On the plus side, if this is possible, I think Crohn's has had a few positive effects on me. For one, it's made me realise what and who is important in my life. BC (before Crohn's), I wasn't a particularly negative person, but I think I was always more inclined to look on the dull side of life. Now I feel so much more positive, and try to cope with my disease by laughing at my misfortune. The thing is, I have Crohn's and there's no getting away from it, so I figure I can either get angry and wallow in the misery of it all, or I can learn to adapt and accept this is now a part of my future.

Crohn's has to be factored into every plan I make, what I eat and drink and it interferes with my social life something terrible. As Crohn's is so unpredictable,

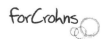

there is no telling how I will feel from one hour to the next, which is very frustrating. It means plans may be cancelled at the last minute and people I care about let down, work missed, or days wasted tucked up in bed –squeezing the cat for dear life (not really, just a wee cuddle). All of that amounts to major disruption in the life of this diseased lady. It's hard to accept that this is my life now, and there's absolutely zilch I can do about it. At times, it feels as if I have no control over my own body.

I manage to cope pretty well with work; I've rarely taken time off in the past few months and I'm getting better at being able to spot the signs of a flare-up. I can usually tell when things are taking a turn for the worse, and try to slow down or cancel plans. It's still a pain in the neck having to worry about these sorts of things, but I'm slowly realising that it must be done. My health has to come first, and I must accept that some things need to take a back seat.

I work in a busy office, so taking breaks or time off is tricky – my bosses and colleagues still *struggle to understand the intricacies of my illness* [2]. I think they still expect things to get steadily worse, which in most cases doesn't happen. An attack or immense pain can happen instantaneously and completely without warning. People are quick to pigeonhole you and assume what may or may not be going on behind the make-up mask. This can be very frustrating when you constantly have to explain your condition

> **2. Lucy (IBD Nurse) says:**
> Both the IBD doctors and nurses can support sufferers in their work environment and if necessary write letters of support to employers explaining the challenges a patient with Crohn's disease faces.

and describe symptoms. It gets boring and irritating, so patience is key!

I've realised who I can rely on for support and who will be by my side when times get tough. My family and friends have been amazing and a constant support from the moment the word "Crohn's" slipped out of my doctor's mouth. I'm all too aware who I can turn to and who will be there for me no matter what. Those who love me have learnt to adapt to me having this disease more easily than I have, and they have helped me through it every step of the way.

I may have had a nasty bit of me removed because of Crohn's, but it's brought out the best in me. I'm stronger for it and I know I'll be able to take on whatever it throws at me in the future. It's very early days with my condition, but I feel I'm going to be OK. Better than OK – things can 'Crohn-ly get better'."

Ruth

Ruth is 55 years old and was diagnosed with Crohn's disease 30 years ago. She is now a part-time bookkeeper and has two children, 26 and 22. Here she talks about how Crohn's impacts her day-to-day life.

"I was diagnosed with Crohn's when I was 25 years old. Although I was very ill during those first few years, when I became pregnant with my first child (Natasha), I had never felt better. Unfortunately it was short-lived. As soon as she was born, my urgent need for the loo resumed. I would often have to knock on strangers' doors to ask to use the toilet and put her on the floor. This was very distressing and humiliating. Even now, I still get embarrassed if I am out with friends, or at their house, and need to go to the loo (going missing for a long time).

My friends all know about my condition, but however much they try and empathise, frankly – unless they suffer in the same way, they really don't know what we go through. A couple of friends have said, after suffering a tummy upset: "I now know what you must feel like". I feel like saying "NO, you don't. You may have one or two days in the loo, but imagine what it is like going 6-7 times a day, every day!"

I try to stay positive and I still lead an active social life, despite my Crohn's. However, it's the small ways that Crohn's impacts your day-to-day life that can get you down. For example, when my son was young, I really wanted to cheer him on when he played football – but heartbreakingly, I never could because of the lack of facilities. When my daughter and I went up for university open days, there were such long queues to get onto the buses that toured accommodation that I had to ask another parent if she minded taking Natasha, while I waited in a café. These situations are really difficult, and I often wish I could lead a "normal life".

People at work also know, but it is never talked about. Thankfully for me, they allow me to work from home two days a week and log-on via a remote desktop connection. This means I now only have to travel into town once a week, which is enough. Getting on a train makes me worry, in case I get stuck in a tunnel. Whenever I do travel on the tube, I keep a printout of the tube map handy – which has all the toilets marked on it, so I know where to get off in case of an emergency. I try to use the Jubilee line where possible, as there are lots of toilets on this line. Sometimes I feel I have to miss out on social events with work because of my

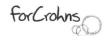

Crohn's. I had to decline a recent outing to France to avoid the embarrassment of my rushing off to find a toilet the whole time.

Travelling abroad can also be difficult [3], and needs some planning ahead and psychological preparation! Firstly, getting to the airport can be a nightmare if there is traffic. Queuing with the cases and needing the loo is dreadful. Then once I'm on the plane, I spend the flight hoping there isn't a queue for the toilets. And when the plane lands, I start to worry about the bus to the terminal. Once in the terminal: "Will there be a loo before going through passport control? Will I be able to explain, if they only speak a foreign language, that I need a loo desperately? How long will the taxi ride to the hotel be? Will it be on the motorway all the way, and will I be able to explain

> **3. Lucy (IBD Nurse) says:**
> Travelling abroad can be difficult with Crohn's disease – there are some useful tips on how to do this via www.ibdpassport.com

they may need to stop?" Despite all these worries, I do enjoy going on holiday and I wouldn't let my Crohn's stop me from having my annual summer break! Once there, I relax and enjoy myself. Similarly, I enjoy going to the theatre, cinema, dining out and I try to push myself out of my comfort zone to ensure I don't miss out on anything – like going to the Emirates to see my favourite team play football!

I now have a gorgeous dog who I love taking for a daily walk. However, this is another aspect of life that can cause anxiety: Will I be able to make it round the block without needing the loo? I have to restrict my route to one local park, where I know they have toilets. Even this will become difficult soon, as they are going to shut them during winter! Thankfully, I have a Radar key, so I can use disabled toilets. I find that having set routines and little tips like the Radar key and tube map helps me stay positive. Quite frankly – you must not let the disease dictate your life, or you would spend all day at home!

Wendy

Wendy is 49, married with one child and works as a writer. She was diagnosed with Crohn's when she was 19, has had many operations and would describe her Crohn's as 'moderate-severe'.
This is Wendy's account of everyday living when you have an ileostomy bag.

"Nobody had told me about leaks. Really. You'd think it would be something someone would give you a little warning about – maybe some kind of pep talk, telling you it happens to everybody and you shouldn't worry when it happens to you, because it will. It's horrible and upsetting, but you just have to be pragmatic about it and remember that it happens to everyone. Everyone with a bag, that is. But nobody did – not the surgeon, not the stoma nurse, not the nice pretty lady with a bag who came to see me before I had mine. None of them.

What you should know is that with Crohn's disease, there's a danger of 'accidents'. The possibility of literally crapping yourself at inopportune moments. That has happened to me. And on more than one occasion. Most memorably when I was recording a radio play at a studio in the centre of London. The studio was in the basement; I was there, watching the actors speak my words, thoughtlessly drinking strong coffee, when suddenly I needed the loo. I needed it urgently. It was up a flight of stairs and round a corner; and as I hurtled up those stairs, I felt the worst happening. By the time I got to the loo, I had to flush away my knickers, wash the top of my jeans and dry them with the hand dryer and then wash my hands about a hundred times. When I'd finished, I then spend the rest of the day swallowing enough Codeine to stop an elephant ever going to the toilet again – convinced I smelled faintly of poo and that everybody was just too polite to mention it. And I couldn't tell anyone – not the actors, not my friend the producer, nobody.

Poo is in its own category when it comes to other peoples'. If someone pees themselves, we mostly feel concern – are they OK? What happened? If a woman's period starts unbeknownst to her and she's wearing white, other women at least will be sympathetic; but if someone has poo on them, we all just recoil in disgust. My teen says "that's because it's disgusting", and that kind of sums it up. In light of this tale, it won't surprise you to know that one of the things I was most excited about when I decided to have a bag, was that I'd never have to deal with a situation like that again. Never. Ever. That was one of the big fat positives that I focused on when I made the decision to have my plumbing rerouted forevermore. To never use the toilet like a 'normal' person ever again. The fact that I would never have to worry about soiling myself in a public arena was a definite plus.

So you can imagine, my first leak, when it happened, was quite a disappointment. It kind of crept up on me, or the realisation of its existence did. I was out shopping with my teen. We were having a laugh; I'd been trying on clothes, for heaven's sake! We were going to stop off for a coffee, but the two places we fancied going were full. It was snowy and cold, so we decided against heading for a third and came back home instead. I sat on his bed, both of us nursing hot drinks, when my hand drifted, as it often does, to my bag area. It was wet. I was confused; had I spilled my hot chocolate? No. Then what on earth… oh shit! Literally. It was a leak.

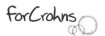

My bag had leaked. How could that be? I dashed to the loo and saw that the side of the bag was coming away, and some of the contents had leaked onto my stomach. I ripped off my leggings, my waistband, my underwear and changed my bag. It wasn't nice, but it was no big deal. And one of the best things about it, compared with my earlier pre-bag experiences, was that the stuff in the bag doesn't smell. I don't know why, but I've had several incidents since then, and it never smells, which is one hell of a positive. Nobody had warned me about this leak thing, but it wasn't the end of the world. At least I was at home, a change of clothes was to hand and it's not like it had gone everywhere. Not that time.

I'm going a bit tangential for a moment now, as I want to talk about showering. There is much debate in the ostomate community about showering – about whether one should shower with a bag or go commando and let the stoma enjoy a bit of running water outside of being cleaned and changed. I liked the idea, but my stoma has no fixed timetable, and the idea of it gushing poo down my leg and into the bath that my family uses is just not something I can handle. So I don't do it. I shower with my bag, though not without feeling a little jealousy towards those who can go commando with impunity.

And so we go back to the stoma, the bag, and the constant element of surprise they bring into my life. Into all of our lives. But never more than the night of the evil early hours leakage. The night that was turning into morning when I woke up to find my bag had completely come away from my skin and all the output (that's what we call it when we're being polite – it's still poo) had done what my worst fears didn't want it ever to do. It was all over me. My pyjamas were covered in it, my stomach was covered in it, and as I leapt up – squealing in horror – it did what gravity dictates it must and started to go all over me. I ran into the bathroom, too horrified even to cry, and stood in the middle of the lino floor, dripping onto it, *unsure of what to do next* [4]. My husband poked his head around the door and said: "Shower. You're going to have to shower". It was 5.30am. I didn't shower at 5.30am unless I was about to have surgery or had an early

4. Phil (Gastro) says:
The amount of 'poo' that comes out of the stoma (the 'output') can vary from person to person and vary depending on the amount of intestine the person has, the food and drink taken in, the disease activity and many other factors. Gastroenterologists can help control this output with medications such as loperamide (Imodium) or tablets that reduce the amount of acid/secretions from the stomach that are produced such as omeprazole. Stoma nurses can also help if 'leakage' appears to become a regular problem with a huge variety of adhesives and bags now available.

flight to catch for a holiday, but what else could I do? This was a huge leak. And... wait a minute. The bag. I couldn't change the bag before I showered; that would be pointless. I couldn't shower with it on because, well... because it was pretty much off. And then realisation dawned – it was 5.30 in the morning; my responses weren't up to speed – I was about to shower commando. So I did. I climbed out of my pooey pjs, disposed of the bag and wiped myself as clean as I could with the usual wipes. I soaked the pooey pjs until they were pooey no more, ran downstairs and shoved them in the washing machine, then ran back up and climbed into the shower. With my stoma out. There I stood, proud of my stomach, pink and innocent, like it could never do anything remotely awful ever. And it didn't while I showered. It behaved and stayed happy and poo-free as I got clean and got dry, and put on a new bag and fresh pyjamas. I have to tell you, it was lovely. Showering properly naked again was a joy. I haven't done it since – I wouldn't dare risk it – but it's the good bit I take away from that horrible experience, and in some ways I don't regret it happening.

I've never slept through the night since then. I always wake up twice to empty my bag – once at about 3am, and again at about 6am. That's what the problem had been; I'd just slept too long and the bag had got too full. I'd actually been out, the night before, for the first time on my own. I'd met up with a bunch of old friends and had a fantastic time – so good that I'd fallen into bed exhausted, and had slept far too soundly – not waking up at all until it was too late. I'd had a wonderful night and a hellish early morning. And if I could only remember the date it happened, I'd designate that Poo Day."

Summary

These stories highlight the many small ways that Crohn's can creep into a person's life on a day-to-day basis and affect small decisions they make. More importantly, they show how these issues can be anticipated, planned for and dealt with so that they are part of a routine. As you've seen, some of the episodes described have been distressing and difficult for those involved, but they include great examples of how to avoid these situations, how to be ready for them and how to deal with them if they occur. They show that while Crohn's will always be a factor in day-to-day life, it doesn't have to control or damage it – in fact these people have taken control themselves and are able to work, travel and lead a normal life.

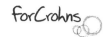

Tips and suggestions

The below come from a range of patients:

- **Get a Radar key**
  This can be obtained from www.radarkeys.org and will allow you to use disabled toilets.

- **Plan ahead/plan your journey**
  Know where toilets are on your route. Have a sense of how long you can go before needing the loo, and plan your journey to give you the best chance of success.

- **Obtain the tube map with toilet information**
  Use toilet links for the tube and others such as 'lootube' (a mobile app).

- **Flexible working**
  Can you arrange to work from home more? Depending on the type of work you do, many employers now offer flexible working arrangements.

- **Use routines to help you, but don't allow them to dictate what you can and can't do.**
  Routines will help you feel comfortable about doing things regularly, but they might make you anxious about anything that alters your routine.

- **Familiarise yourself with your surroundings**
  Or the surroundings of where you're going – it's worth scoping out the facilities when you arrive somewhere and have an exit strategy, just in case.

- **Plan ahead if possible**
  Try and recognise signs of a flare-up and cancel plans.

- **Use any practical tools at your disposal**
  Get hold of the Crohn's and Colitis UK Can't Wait card. This card will help you to be able to use a toilet in an emergency. It also comes in foreign languages.

Keep 20p and 50p coins handy in case you need the loo in city centres or on the tube.

Get letters from the places you go frequently to show you have permission to use the disabled loo if it doesn't have a Radar lock.

- **Be aware of where toilets are on long journeys**
  Make sure you have petrol stations, hotels and supermarkets visible on sat navs, as they are often open 24 hours and are the easiest places to go if you need the loo urgently.
  Check online where all service stations are for when you're on a long journey.

- **Carry spare underwear, wet wipes and tissues.**
  Accidents happen and it is always best to be prepared. Tissues are also an essential for when you enter a public toilet with no loo paper.

- **Jelly Babies can be a tasty (if slightly unhealthy) alternative to loperamide.**
  Two Jelly Babies are equivalent to taking one Loperamide. A nice sweet treat after lunch!

- **When you are out and about, think carefully about the food you eat**.
  It's fairly obvious that if you eat something hot and spicy, you might need the toilet a lot that afternoon. Just be wary of the consequences of what you eat.

- **Exercise your pelvic floor muscles.**
  Don't always give in to every temptation to go to the loo (this is best practiced at home). One tip is to put a chair outside the bathroom. When you feel you really need to go to the loo, walk to the bathroom, sit on the chair (facing away from the toilet), and count slowly to ten, clenching your bum muscles. Then stand up and see if you still need the toilet. If you do – then go, you don't want an accident. But often you'll find you don't. Give it a try!

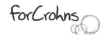

- **Make sure you plan some toilet visits.**
  If you know you are going to be on transport for an hour, make sure you go to the loo before you leave the house, even if you don't feel you need to. If you have been out for dinner and are about to leave a restaurant, go to the loo. It is better to avoid a blind panic on the way home.

- **Starving yourself won't stop you from going to the loo.**
  In fact, it might make things worse. On days that you feel bad, try and eat something, even if it's dry toast/crackers.

- **Ileostomy bag – it will leak at some point!**
  It's ok, it happens to everyone occasionally. Your stoma nurse may be able to help improve things and get the best fitting appliance possible, but always carry plenty of spares and clean up stuff. A quickly cleaned up leak will not become a talking point.

- **Change your bag during the night to avoid it getting too full.**
  If your output is very loose, then night-time bags with a tube to a larger reservoir by the side of the bed may mean a longer night's sleep. Discuss this with your stoma nurse.

- **Loperamide or codeine can be used in various doses.**
  You might want to avoid taking large doses most of the time, but if you're going to a wedding (for example), those extra couple of tablets might give you a bit more confidence for the first few hours of the day. Don't forget that loperamide is best taken 30 minutes to one hour before food.

- **Don't let Crohn's rule your life**
  Don't let your Crohn's get in the way of your activities – you can still live your life.

- **You are not alone**
  Talk to friends, family, your IBD nurse, people with Crohn's online or sign up to the forCrohns buddy scheme.

Drugs used in Crohn's disease

Medication plays a large role in the management of Crohn's disease. Most people diagnosed with Crohn's will have to take different types of medication, and since drugs work differently in different people, it's important to understand the risks and benefits of each drug before using them. This chapter explains the various types of drugs and the experiences of different patients using them in reality. The trials that assess how effective drugs are and also identify their side effects are published in countless scientific papers. The most important data from such studies are reviewed and collected by experts in IBD as reviews or in books. An example is 'Inflammatory Bowel Disease, An Evidence-based Practical Guide'. It is a medical book designed for healthcare professionals who treat people with Crohn's and UC, edited by Dr Ailsa Hart and Dr Siew Ng, who are IBD experts. The authors have collected and reviewed the medical literature on managing IBD from around the world.

Crohn's disease from the medics

Drugs for Crohn's disease

There are many different drugs used in Crohn's disease, and new drugs appear on a regular basis. As discussed in section 1, the exact cause of Crohn's disease is not known, and as a result, most of the drugs used tend to reduce inflammation (anti-inflammatories) or dampen the action of the immune system (immunosuppressants or immunomodulators). It is often unclear what specific

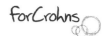

effects various drugs have, but clinical trials have been used to determine which drugs are useful in which circumstances. Guidelines produced by organisations like the BSG (British Society of Gastroenterology) and ECCO (European Crohn's and Colitis Organisation) are designed to keep care fairly consistent around the country and give patients good treatment based on the best evidence available.

The range of disease in Crohn's is quite large. Some people just get a bit of diarrhoea, which is controlled using drugs like Loperamide or Codeine, which simply thicken the stool (poo) and make you need to go less often. More severe symptoms may require more powerful drugs.

What are the different drugs in Crohn's disease and how do they work?

Steroids

When inflammation is more severe, steroids may be needed to get an acute attack under control. Steroids are powerful and effective, and can be given by mouth or into the vein, which makes them very useful. However, they have side-effects, which can be severe if taken for long periods. These include weight-gain, thinning of the skin, osteoporosis (thinning of the bone), the face becoming round, stretch marks and many others. These side-effects are not a problem when steroids are used for short periods, and they are very effective at reducing inflammation. If steroids have been used for more than a few days, they need to be reduced gradually rather than stopped abruptly, because the body can become reliant on them and stop producing the natural steroid hormones it needs. The steroids must then be stopped slowly (weaned) so the body has a chance to start producing these 'endogenous' (meaning produced within the patient's body) steroids again.

Immunosuppressants

After steroids have 'induced remission' (made the patient well again), patients will often be switched onto a different type of drug to maintain this remission. Azathioprine or Mercaptopurine are often used and dampen the immune system, which can keep patients well for long periods. Some people cannot tolerate these drugs and for others, they simply don't work. A blood test (called TPMT) is taken when azathioprine is prescribed, which can help determine whether it will be useful in that person.

Other immunosuppressant drugs include Cyclosporine, methotrexate and Thalidomide. These drugs are often used when other treatments have failed and can have serious side-effects, but they do also work very well in some patients. They are never prescribed in pregnancy.

If the colon, or in particular, the rectum is affected, another type of drug called a 5-ASA is used – for example mesalazine, which can be given as a tablet or, if the inflammation is in the rectum, as a suppository or enema (a tablet or liquid that is put into the bottom). Antibiotics such as metronidazole are also often used in combination with other drug treatments.

Anti TNF alpha drugs

Newer drugs such as infliximab and adalimumab (Remicade and Humira are examples of trade names for them) are able to improve patients' symptoms and induce healing in the bowel. They are also able to treat some fistulas (tunnels of infection, see section 1), especially anal, abdominal or rectovaginal fistulas, much more effectively than the other drugs mentioned above. They are expensive and have some serious side-effects, which your doctor will discuss with you if they plan to offer you these drugs, but they can be extremely effective even when other treatments have failed. They are thought to work by interfering with a particular cytokine, TNF alpha, which is one of the chemicals used by your immune system to encourage inflammation. They are given by injection, either every two months into the vein by a nurse (infliximab), or fortnightly into the skin (adalimumab), which most patients are able to do themselves, at home.

New drugs, currently in clinical trials before being licensed, interfere with different cytokines and both doctors and patients are keen to know just how well these new drugs will work.

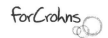

Type of Drug	Examples	Mechanism of action	Side-effects
Antibiotics	Metronidazole	Kill bacteria which might be driving inflammation	Few, mostly mild
Steroids	Prednisolone, Hydrocortisone	Reduce inflammation	Significant, particularly if taken for long periods
Anti-inflammatory drugs	5-ASA, Mesalazine	Reduce inflammation	Mostly mild
Immunosuppressants	Azathioprine, 6MP	Depress the immune system	Some are intolerant of these drugs
Anti TNF agents	Infliximab, Adalimumab	Block TNF alpha activity and reduce inflammation	Unusual but can be severe
Others	Cyclosporin, Methotrexate, Thalidomide	Various	Often very significant side-effects, so these drugs are not often used

Figure 2. Drugs used in Crohn's disease

Dietary treatments

Special diets such as elemental diets and FODMAP diets can also produce improvement in patient's symptoms. These are discussed in the following chapter on diet and nutrition.

Surgery

Sometimes, medicines will not make patients better. For example, strictures (narrowing), abscesses or some types of fistula (tunnel of infection) often require surgery because no medical treatment will help. Sometimes medical treatment fails for reasons we don't understand, and patients continue to deteriorate despite best treatment, or are so unwell that it is not safe to wait for medical treatment to work. In these situations too, surgery is needed to protect the patient from harm, reduce symptoms and induce remission. After surgery, drugs such as azathioprine may again be used to try and maintain the remission for as long as possible.

Probiotics

Although the exact cause of Crohn's is not known, a change to the normal bacteria of the gut is thought to be involved. As a result, probiotics (which may make the bacteria in the gut return to a more normal state) are often used by patients, although rarely prescribed by their doctor. The idea is that if the probiotics make your gut bacteria normal, there may be less inflammation in the gut. Unfortunately, there is no evidence from clinical trials that probiotics are effective in Crohn's disease. Most of the trials are small and it is possible that as more trials are performed or new probiotics come on the market, a benefit may be found, but at the moment it is not possible to say that probiotics will help patients with Crohn's disease.

Complementary medicine

Many patients use complementary medicine treatments such as homeopathy, naturopathy, acupuncture and herbal medicines, and find real benefit in these alternative therapies. The use of these treatments has increased dramatically in recent decades, and a half of patients asked in some scientific studies say they use them. Patients often say they decided to try complementary medicines because of the side-effects caused by conventional treatments – they feel there are fewer side-effects to complementary treatments, or that doing so gives them more control over their disease. Unfortunately, patients using complementary medicines do not always discuss this with their doctor, which puts them at risk of interactions, meaning that the complementary medicines they take can reduce the effectiveness of conventional medicines or lead to dangerous side-effects. Although complementary medicines are thought of as 'natural' and therefore safer than conventional medicines, serious side-effects such as liver or kidney damage can occasionally occur.

Most importantly, there is almost no scientific evidence that complementary therapies benefit those with Crohn's disease. It is difficult to undertake scientific research in complementary treatments, so it may be that western science is simply unable to detect the benefits of complementary medicines, and certainly some patients claim that complementary therapies have improved their lives dramatically. If a Crohn's patient is considering using complementary medicines, they should discuss this with their doctor, so that any interaction with conventional medicines can be avoided.

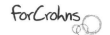

Nutritional supplements

Crohn's can often lead to poor nutrition, either because the bowel is too inflamed to allow absorption, or because important sections of the bowel have been removed at surgery. Some of the drugs used may also mean that taking nutritional supplements is wise. Calcium, vitamins D and B12, iron, folate and others may all be low, and your doctor may recommend taking supplements to boost your levels of these.

Summary

There are several drugs used in the treatment of Crohn's disease. Whenever you start a new drug, your doctor or IBD Nurse will discuss the likelihood of benefit and any potential risks, so you can decide whether or not you want to try it. The success of medical treatment in Crohn's can be very variable; some patients may use one or two drugs over long periods with good results, whereas others may end up switching between different drugs every few months because of a lack of results. With any drug treatment, try to analyse whether you are gaining a benefit, look out for side-effects that seem related to any new drug you take, and be patient – sometimes several weeks of treatment are required to see the effectiveness of a drug.

Crohn's disease from the patients

The following section looks at the experience of five people who have had medication for Crohn's disease. Everyone's experience is different because people respond to drugs in different ways, but this section will hopefully answer a few questions about the reality of taking medications and the improvements and effects they can have.

55

Louise

Louise is 24 years old and works as a shop assistant. She describes her Crohn's as quite severe and was diagnosed a little under two years ago. Here she discusses some of her experiences with steroids, azathioprine and Humira.

"When it comes to medicating Crohn's, the NHS takes a pyramid outlook. *They start at the bottom with the standard round of drugs and treatments that control inflammation*[1]. If these fail, they move up the scale of medications, to ones that are stronger and have more serious side-effects. Then they move into biological treatments that are costly and have higher risk factors. Then, the option becomes surgery. The last option – cut out the bad bowel and reduce the inflammation.

I was given the first round of Crohn's medication in early September 2011. Prednisolone – steroids, the most basic level of medication to reduce inflammation in the bowels; Pentasa – an anti-inflammation drug for mild to moderate Crohn's and Colitis, and Adcal – calcium tablets that must be taken alongside Prednisolone to avoid *bone deterioration*[2]. I spent two weeks on these tablets – a daily 40mg of pred, three Adcal and 2g of Pentasa. It was tough going and I have terrible memories of trying to take *eight Pentasa tablets twice a day*[3].

1. Phil (Gastro) says:
This is certainly one approach for those who present with milder disease, but whose disease progresses. However, the severity of disease, its location and behaviour will all influence this decision ultimately. Discuss it with your gastroenterologist if you are not sure.

2. Phil (Gastro):
All patients with IBD should have a test called a DEXA scan to look at their bone density, especially if they have been on long term steroids.

3. Lucy (IBD Nurse):
There are lots of preparations of these types of anti-inflammatory medications (5-ASA) to reduce the 'pill burden' massively

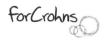

By the time I was seen by my consultant, this course of treatment wasn't helping my inflammation. I spent two weeks in the Gastro ward – where I *caught C Diff* [4] for the first time – and they considered more options. Here they discussed their desire to avoid surgery at all costs and told me I could get funding for a biological treatment – *either Remicade or Humira* [5] – and this would be administered when things got to the 'severe' category. The fact that I could get so sick that I'd need a very strong drug to keep me healthy was scary. I sat with my IBD nurses on the ward as they talked me through the process, and when this would become my fate, if at all. In the same discussion, I was introduced to something called azathioprine – an *immunosuppressant drug* [6] used in organ transplants and could maintain clinical remission of Crohn's disease. I was in shock. I had only been a Crohn's sufferer for just over a month, and already I'd been in twice with symptoms. I was caught between wanting to get better and being so scared things would get so bad that I'd need the surgery sooner than planned. I was worried, and hardly slept during this admission. Reluctantly, I was started on this after my antibiotics – metronidazole and Vancomycin – for my C Diff in mid-October.

During one clinic appointment a couple of weeks later, the consultant upped my azathioprine from 50 to 100mg daily. It didn't help, I was in hospital a day later. My Crohn's had gotten worse. I was now considered to have severe Crohn's disease. It was time for the biological treatments.

I started *Humira* in early December, after finishing more rounds of antibiotics and putting some weight on. I have remained on a 40mg bi-weekly dose since January of this year.

4. Phil (Surgeon) says:
Clostridium Difficile is a bacteria which can affect the bowel causing inflammation. It is usually treated with antibiotics but occasionally surgery is needed. It is not specifically related to Crohn's disease but it tends to occur in hospitals in people who are already ill in some other way.

5. Phil (Gastro):
Adalimumab (Humira) is a drug similar to Infliximab (Remicade) and known to induce healing in some Crohn's patients. It is one of the more recent biological drugs that has become available to patients with IBD. Before starting this medication, patients will need to be screened for TB and viruses that cause hepatitis (liver inflammation) before starting.

6. Lucy (IBD Nurse):
When starting patients on powerful immunosuppression patients are always counselled as to the benefits but also the risks medications. Patients often need to be monitored whilst on these medications (e.g. blood tests) and may need screening for any pre-existing conditions or infections prior to starting treatments.

Injecting myself in the thigh every other Thursday hasn't always been a walk in the park. To begin with, I was supervised in the hospital for administering it. Once I got home, I applied the gusto I'd had to get through my admissions to my medication routine. I went back to work and continued to feel better, and returned to an almost normal life – a Crohnie life with very few problems and symptoms.

It came to April and everything changed. I don't even know what had changed, nor what triggered my anxiety, but I couldn't do my injections anymore. I was terrified of the needle. I was also very aware that I was better and didn't need this every other Thursday. But of course, I did, I was just stupid enough to think I was smarter. I'm not, so I got in contact with my IBD nurse and we did them together at the hospital for a couple rounds. Now? I'm back to doing them at home. I wouldn't have known what to do – about most things to do with my medications and symptoms – without the IBD nurse. Every time something new is added or something changes, she is first on my list to call. I can't always get out of work or get to an emergency GI clinic appointment, so her answer phone system has kept me sane many times over.

I always did my own research into the full extent of my medication list. I always made sure I was discharged with all my notes and lists of medications. *I always questioned the junior doctors about the orders; in fact I could be quite annoying and insistent* [7]. *I was always eager for ward rounds and didn't stop finding out what was going on with my care.* I would rather know the bullet than have something sprung upon me. Please always ask questions, even if they are simple and silly and they bug you throughout the day or night. Doctors are there to answer your questions before they proceed with your course of treatment. Don't assume that everything you are having done is for the best, get involved. Be your own advocate."

7. Phil (Gastro) and Phil (Surgeon) say:
Doctors often find it much easier to care for patients who take ownership of their illness and are involved in their own care. It is not annoying and if you don't understand why you are on something or what it is then the explanations you have been given are inadequate, so always ask until you're clear. Your IBD nurse may well be able to fill in the gaps for you too.

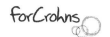

Deepan

Deepan is 23 and is currently studying childcare. Here he discusses some of his experiences with steroids and azathioprine.

"When taking steroids for the first time, my face blew up like a blowfish [8]*.* I started eating like an animal and developed a pot belly! My bones became brittle and I was getting joint pains often. This, I understood, was a permanent consequence of taking the steroids, as it diminishes the strength of the joints and you can develop Osteoarthritis. The only tips I can think of when taking medication are: firstly, liquid versions leave a bad taste in your mouth, and pills go down without any taste. Secondly, try not to forget your medication – it might start off as a day missed here or there, and you think nothing of it, but then a day becomes days, weeks or even months at a time. Before long, you'll go into relapse and realise it's because you 'forgot' your medication.

I never saw any side-effects for Azathioprine, other than being susceptible to infections. *Thalidomide* [9], I was told, can make any children I father have physical deformities – but luckily I didn't have to worry about that. Apart from those, I was very fortunate to suffer very few side-effects, apart from small scars from all the blood tests, and infusion sites – but that's to be expected."

8. Phil (Gastro):
Patients can put on weight and their face can become more rounded – a 'moonface'. These are some of the classic side-effects of steroids and they are well recognised. Many of these problems reverse once the steroids are stopped.

9. Phil (Surgeon) says:
You may have heard of Thalidomide which, when it was first introduced for other reasons many years ago, led to physical deformities of children born to parents who had been taking the drug. Before Thalidomide is prescribed this will be very carefully discussed with you so you can avoid becoming pregnant or fathering a child until well after you have stopped taking it when doing so becomes safe once again.

Will

Will is 33 and married with two kids. He was diagnosed aged 16, and now works as a web development consultant. Here he discusses his experiences of steroids, azathioprine and changing his diet.

"Just before my final-year exams at school, I became really ill. I had not been very well for a while, but it was getting serious now and my weight was plummeting. My appetite was non-existent and I found it hard to keep food down.

The doctors kept diagnosing me with colic, and sending me home with ineffective medication. It got so bad one day that my mother phoned up the hospital and told them to prepare a bed for me. So after numerous trips to the doctor, I was finally admitted to hospital. When I arrived I was left in a wheelchair with a cardboard bowl to be sick in.

Luckily, my mum had been pretty insistent. Something wasn't right and she managed to get me an appointment with an expert in gastroenterology. I was then admitted to my local hospital and treated by a gastroenterologist – who has now been looking after me for 13 years, and proven to be a true expert in her field.

After being admitted to hospital, I was finally diagnosed with Crohn's disease. It was a relief to be labelled with a condition, as treatment could begin. It was frightening not knowing what was happening to me; at 16, my weight was under seven stone and I had no strength. My parents were also strangely delighted with the diagnosis, as they had feared the worst and thought I had childhood cancer.

Treatment began. Initially I was put on steroids – I preferred the little red sugar-coated ones, *as they didn't taste bitter*[10]. Thankfully, the medication was very effective. The only downside was that the steroids were very harsh. I would sweat profusely and wake up in the middle of the night with the worst cramp in unimaginable places, and had to

> **10. Phil (Surgeon) says:**
> This is the most common oral steroid used in Crohn's disease. It is probably the same drug that Will was given in the first place but a different type and strength of tablet. Various formulations are often available of each drug and if you're not getting on with one be specific about what you don't like so that your doctors can try the same drug in a different form if that's what you need.

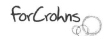

suffer chubby red cheeks. Not great side-effects – but I was thankful that recovery had begun.

I was also given *prednisolone, which I believed to be an anti-inflammatory drug, but I now understand it is a Corticosteroid.* These were huge pills that had little flakes of the drug suspended in a white solid powder, which made them really hard to swallow. I regularly gagged – not a nice experience.

It took me a while to get over this low point. Putting on weight was extremely difficult. I was given all manner of disgusting weight-gain drinks and an experimental Nestle branded powder-based product, which was tolerable.

Eventually, I came off the steroids and started taking azathioprine. The azathioprine was a revelation. This drug is an immune suppressant and was relatively new at the time; but it seems I was one of the lucky ones who reacted positively to it. It meant that I was able to come off of the steroids and avoid the horrible side-effects. The medical team were keen on monitoring the drug's effects on my body, so I had to go in for regular blood tests. As it transpires, after years of taking azathioprine, it seems to be relatively safe and I did not suffer any notable side-effects.

I would still get really fatigued and feel constantly tired when I got home from college. After some blood tests, I was found to be *anaemic* [11], for which I was given folic acid and shots of vitamin B12 in the arm, which helped a bit.

For a few years, I was on and off medication. I would stop taking azathioprine, and after a few months the symptoms of Crohn's would creep back.

My aunty then put me *on the York test* [12] – a simple blood intolerance test. I must say, I was sceptical, as the test was not cheap and it was not officially recognised by the medical profession as a proven method of diagnosis. Luckily, my generous aunty offered to pay for a test, and the results returned a high intolerance to yeast.

11. Phil (Surgeon) says:
Lots of people with Crohn's are anaemic at some point in their lives. This may be related to inflammation or removal of an important stretch of the bowel which absorbs some crucial substances like vitamin B12.

12. Phil (Gastro):
This test is not used in routine medical practice as there is no clear and independent evidence for its use.

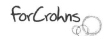

In hindsight, this really made sense and I changed my diet accordingly. This made a *massive difference* [13] and I felt immensely better. To this day I avoid yeast products, bread, beer, wine, pastries, Oxo cubes, Marmite – the list goes on. It was quite a challenge at first, as the Western diet revolves around breaded goods.

Despite all this, I still had bouts of Crohn's and only fully felt better when I followed the advice of the doctors and stopped smoking. *I cannot stress the importance of this enough!* [14]

I am now finally off medication after 13 years, and in remission. My tips for combatting Crohn's, in order of importance, would be: do not smoke, take note of foods that do not agree with you, have a healthy balanced diet, do not drink too much alcohol, stay active and try not to get too stressed. Basically – look after yourself.

Do not be afraid to ask questions of your doctors and seek a second opinion.

I consider myself lucky, as I only suffered moderate Crohn's disease and have managed to control it and get on with my life. Hopefully new treatments, like infliximab, will continue to prove effective in combatting Crohn's disease and the illness will prove less debilitating for others in future. Best wishes to my fellow Crohn's sufferers."

This chapter will now explore some complementary therapies

13. Phil (Gastro) and Phil (Surgeon) say:
It is difficult to explain this in the context of Crohn's disease. Certainly some foods affect some patients more than others and food intolerances can exist alongside Crohn's disease as they can in anyone else. It is sensible for any Crohn's sufferer to be aware of their reaction to any specific food or food group and discuss this with their gastroenterologist.

14. Phil (Gastro) and Phil (Surgeon) say:
Stopping smoking is probably the most important single step an individual can take to help their Crohn's disease. Time and again studies have shown that smoking increases the severity of Crohn's disease, the risk of flares and the chance of requiring surgery. Seriously, give up smoking.

Complementary and alternative medicine includes a wide range of practices and therapies outside the realms of conventional western medicine.

Despite a lack of scientific data in the form of controlled trials, for either effectiveness or safety of complementary and alternative medicine, the use by patients with inflammatory bowel disease, particularly of herbal therapies, is widespread and increasing.

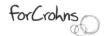

There is limited controlled evidence that indicates effectiveness of traditional Chinese medicines, aloe vera gel, wheat grass juice, Boswellia serrata and bovine colostrum enemas in Ulcerative Colitis. Encouraging results have been reported in small studies of acupuncture for Crohn's disease and Ulcerative Colitis. Contrary to popular belief, natural therapies are not necessarily safe: fatal hepatic and irreversible renal failure have occurred with some preparations, and interactions with conventional drugs are potentially dangerous so it is always important to tell your doctors and nurses what additional therapies you are taking.

There is a need for further controlled clinical trials of the effectiveness of complementary and alternative approaches in inflammatory bowel disease, together with enhanced legislation to maximise their quality and safety.

Sue

Sue is 59 and has had Crohn's disease for over 30 years. Here she talks of her experience with homeopathy and acupuncture.

> **15. Phil (Surgeon) says:**
> Fascinating that Sue disregards the possibility that it is these medicines which are helping but rather assumes it must be the homeopathy despite taking them both at the same time.

"Approximately 31 years ago, after my operation in 1976, I had severe arthritis in my whole body from my neck down. This was associated with Crohn's, and I was put on a large dose of steroids, which helped the pain, but had other side-effects. I couldn't continue with them, and someone suggested acupuncture – within six months, I was free of pain.

Approximately 20 years ago, I had another bout of severe pain from Crohn's, and someone suggested homeopathy. I had no recommendation and just picked a lady's name out of a directory, as she lived close to me. As I didn't like the side-effects from the various drugs, I had nothing to lose. I realised that homeopathy would not cure my Crohn's, but I thought it would make my life more bearable, and over time, that is what it's done. I have been seeing someone for the past 20 years every one/two months and *have rarely experienced any side-effects* [15].

In these appointments, you talk to them about the emotional side as well as your physical problems; from relationships, to work, to you as a person, your character etc. You have to be quite honest, as they look at the whole picture, and that is what they treat – it isn't just a pill to pop for helping your stomach, but a pill that incorporates the stomach as well as you as a person. For example, as I help others (perhaps sometimes to the detriment of my wellbeing), my homeopath sees me as a "caretaker" and takes this into consideration. My immune system is not good, so in the past, the treatment has helped me with glandular fever, shingles, depression, hot flushes, and chest infections *as well as the Crohn's*. Despite this, my homeopath *is happy that I continue to take conventional medicine and has never tried to stop me* [16]."

> **16. Phil (Gastro) says:**
> This is very important. Advice to stop taking the kinds of powerful drugs used in Crohn's disease should come from your doctors since stopping them abruptly can in some cases be dangerous.

Tara

Tara is 42 and married with two kids. She was diagnosed at 23 and has had one operation. Here she talks about her experience with yoga and reflexology.

"I've had Crohn's disease for over 20 years, so it's rather a long time ago that I started on the alternative route. To begin with, I didn't really suffer with diarrhoea, but constipation and blockages due to strictures.

I remember going to a local Chinese herbal shop. It was quite farcical. I couldn't understand her and I have no idea if she understood me either! Unfortunately, she thought I suffered with diarrhoea and gave me these enormous golf ball objects that I had to crack open and eat! OMG! They were hideous, disgusting, vomit-inducing and the most evil substance I have ever placed in my mouth! I did try a few times, in the hope that I would become accustomed to them and they might help, but all they did was make me more constipated. I was also given ginseng for more energy, but that sadly lacked too.

Then I tried a naturopath. Lots of money for some advice, but I gave up due to the cost and boredom! It did make me review my diet, which was carb-heavy, but I lost the will and finances to continue.

Next on the list was reflexology. This was an amazing experience. I have an open mind when it comes to alternative therapies; if it works, then fantastic, even if it is only a placebo effect – but how on earth does your body relate to certain points in your feet? I don't know! All I do know is that when Susan (my friend and reflexologist) massages the points on my feet that correlate to my intestines, they

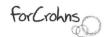

respond with a loud and emphatic grumble! I find it incredibly relaxing and maybe that is part of the therapy too. My stress levels being too high can only aggravate my Crohn's, so this alleviates some of the stress.

I have also attended a yoga class for over 10 years. Again, as with anything, you have to find a class and teacher who suit your needs, and I am lucky to have found a few over the years. I endeavour to do some yoga every day, but consistency and self-control aren't my strong points! However, I find it incredibly relaxing. For an hour and a half, I can eventually switch my whirring brain off and put my mind, body and spirit back into alignment. Some weeks are better than others! In fact, I love yoga so much and find it so beneficial, that I think everyone should practice it, regardless of any health issues.

> **17. Phil (Gastro):**
> Complimentary therapy has an important place in treating the 'whole person' with Crohn's disease. Whilst taking homeopathic remedies may not be recommended (because there is no evidence for them and there is the possibility they could make you unwell in the long term), therapies such as reflexology are harmless and reducing stress in Crohn's patients is very valuable.

It is calming, relaxing, restoring and rejuvenating. I have dragged myself to a class when I have felt so bloated, sore and ill, yet always come out feeling better. I may still be sore and feeling battered, but something has shifted and changed. An early night with a hot water bottle, and I feel somewhat restored the next day. I think it is all the negative thoughts and feelings that get dispersed which calm your head and body. So your illness hasn't gone, you are not miraculously cured, but you have helped to heal yourself (even a little) by *attending a yoga class*." [17]

Summary

Everyone has their own experience of various drugs. For some people, a particular drug is a wonderful saviour, and for someone else, that same drug will be ineffective or worse – lead to side-effects that make them feel ill. It's sensible to keep an open mind about any drugs you haven't tried before and also remember that drugs sometimes work better in combination, even if they haven't been too effective on their own. Other (holistic) treatments can also be valuable for some people, and many patients find that these help them to feel more in control of their bodies and cope with the difficulties Crohn's throws at them. It is always worth discussing changes to your drug regime – what are you trying to achieve? What are the likely side-effects? When can you expect to see a response?

Most people find a particular drug or set of drugs that ultimately keep them free of symptoms or under control for long periods, and this is the aim of the medical treatment of Crohn's.

Tips and suggestions

The following tips and suggestions are taken from our contributors' (patients and healthcare professionals) experiences of different medicated treatments.

- **Don't suddenly stop your medication**
  Always talk to your doctor before changing or stopping a drug (especially steroids), unless you appear to be having a reaction to it – such as a rash or difficulty in breathing.

- **Discuss complementary medicine with your doctor**
  If you are going to use any complementary medicine, discuss this with your doctor to avoid dangerous interactions.

- **Try not to forget to take your medicine**
  Get into the habit of taking your medicine at the same time each day so it becomes a habit.

- **Make sure you know what to expect from your medication**
  Discuss any new drug with your doctor in detail so you know what to expect and what side-effects to watch out for.

- **Keep a diary of how the drug affects you**
  Keep a diary of your symptoms and side-effects so that even a subtle change can be detected.

Having surgery

Unfortunately, the majority of Crohn's patients are likely to undergo surgery at some point in their lives. The aim of that surgery is to reduce the symptoms and suffering from Crohn's. While we know that it is a scary and difficult time, we believe that having an understanding of what the procedures are likely to involve will help you cope. This chapter combines an explanation of the different types of surgery (explained in layman's terms by a surgeon) with genuine patient stories from those who have undergone surgery – the reality of the experience, how they dealt with surgery, and ultimately, the difference it made to their lives.

Crohn's disease from the medics

Use of surgery

Surgery in Crohn's disease used to be mainly undertaken after complications, such as a narrowing or fistula, had occurred. Increasingly, it is believed that an early operation can help to prevent these complications and achieve longer-lasting control of the disease from an earlier stage. Surgery can often greatly improve a person's quality of life.

Fast facts – surgery

- Many Crohn's sufferers, perhaps up to 80 per cent, will undergo surgery of some kind during their lives.

- Surgery does not cure Crohn's disease, but it is designed to either treat a complication (like a fistula or stricture), or to prevent them.

- After surgery, the problems the operation treated can return, but some people experience long periods of remission.

- Generally speaking, surgery for Crohn's disease is either on the abdomen (to remove an inflamed section of intestine or to remove or widen bits of intestine with fistulas or strictures), or around the back passage (to treat fistulas or other problems in this area).

- A stoma (colostomy or ileostomy bag) is sometimes necessary for safety and can provide a better period of relief from symptoms, but it is not always needed and is often temporary when it is used.

- Your surgeon will carry out an operation only after full discussion of all the appropriate and feasible options – they will not force anyone into surgery, nor will they try to do extra surgery that a patient has refused. Increasingly, the advice a surgeon offers about which operation is best comes from a multidisciplinary team made up of surgeons, gastroenterologists, radiologists and other specialists.

- Major surgery always has a long recovery time, and this is particularly true in people who are underweight or already ill, such as those suffering from active Crohn's disease before the operation.

- Healing after surgery can be slow for Crohn's sufferers. This means a longer recovery time and sometimes a slowly-healing wound which might need dressings or other care for longer than you might find in people without Crohn's.

- If you're going to undergo surgery, take time to discuss it with your surgeon and understand what it's for, what it will achieve and what you can expect during your recovery.

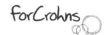

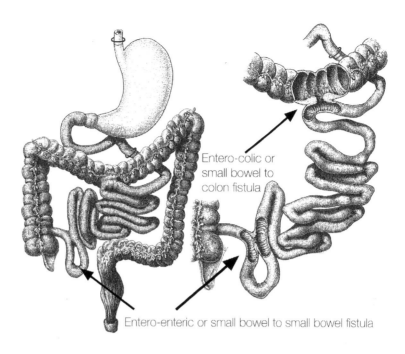

Entero-colic or
small bowel to
colon fistula

Entero-enteric or small bowel to small bowel fistula

Figure 4. Fistulas between different parts of the bowel

Types of surgery

There are different types of surgery for people with Crohn's disease. The following are examples of the more common operations undertaken:

When undertaking surgery on patients with Crohn's the aim to remove as little bowel as possible but to remove or repair diseased segments of bowel, which may be in the small or large bowel. Your surgeon will discuss the plan for the operation you need which may involve removal of some sections of bowel, repair (stricturoplasty, for example – see below) of others and may mean surgery to several parts of the bowel at once. Rather than try to explain each different possible type of operation we have given some examples below. The key is to have a careful discussion with your surgeon before and after your operation to understand exactly what is planned and what has happened.

Right hemicolectomy or ileocolic resection

One common operation is called '**right hemicolectomy**'. This means removal of the right-hand side of the large bowel (colon), along with part of the small bowel (ileum) where it joins the colon. This is the most commonly affected area of the bowel in Crohn's disease and there is usually inflammation (a hot, red, ulcerated, painful area) but also sometimes a narrowing (stricture). This section of bowel is either removed by keyhole surgery or with a cut in the middle of the abdomen, and the two ends are usually joined back together (anastomosis). The operation sometimes needs to be repeated as Crohn's disease can recur at the site of a join – so the amount of bowel removed will always be as small as possible, sometimes only a few inches, and is often called 'ileocaecal or ileocolic resection' instead of the formal 'right hemicolectomy'.

The terminal ileum and right colon are removed.
The remaining ends can be joined together with staples or stitches.

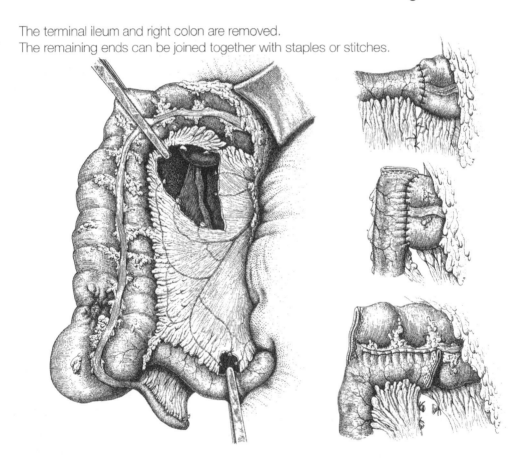

Figure 5. Right hemicolectomy

Stoma

When a join is unwise or impossible, usually because there is a high risk that any join made would leak, a **stoma** can be brought out. These stomas may be

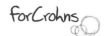

temporary to allow an area of bowel (such as a join) to heal. Your surgeon will explain the reason for making a stoma and whether it can be reversed (to get rid of the stoma) in the future.

Stoma means 'mouth', because the end of the bowel is brought to the skin of the abdomen like an open mouth. Waste comes out of the bowel and into a stoma bag, where it is safely stored until the bag is emptied into a toilet. There are two types of stoma commonly used in Crohn's disease: an **ileostomy and a colostomy**. Ileostomies stick out a few centimetres from the skin in a 'spout', which protects the skin from the digestive enzymes present in the waste from the ileum.

A colostomy produces only faeces, which is not harmful to the skin, so no spout is needed and the stoma does not stick out at all. In both cases, the stoma is easily hidden beneath clothes so that no one will know you have one, and a well-fitted bag does not leak or allow smells to escape.

Stoma nurses

These are a special group of nurses who are highly trained and specifically look after patients with stomas. They will see you before surgery (except in the most dire of emergencies) and again afterwards to give you information and support. They will show you how to look after your stoma and train you in cleaning, emptying, changing it and so on. They can continue to see you after your surgery for as long as you need, and can offer great advice, support and information.

Stricturoplasty

Sometimes narrowings appear elsewhere in the small bowel. Surgeons generally try to avoid removing bowel in Crohn's patients, as repeated flare-ups and operations to remove sections can lead to problems with too little bowel surface left to absorb nutrients. An alternative when dealing with narrowings that are quite short is a **stricturoplasty**. This involves cutting the narrowed part of the bowel long ways and then sewing it up across ways so the section of bowel is widened but shortened. The surface area, which is the important bit for absorption of nutrients from the food, is unchanged in this operation.

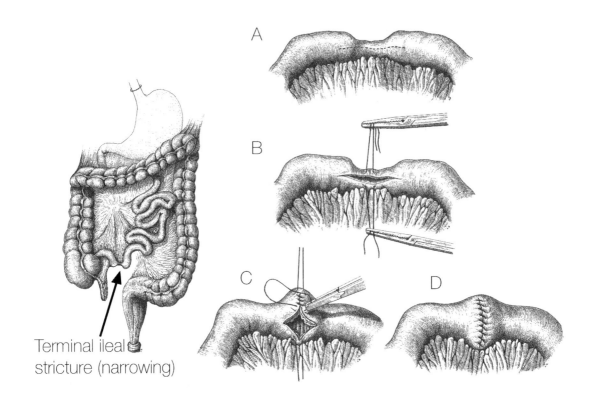

Terminal ileal stricture (narrowing)

Figure 6. A stricture in the terminal ileum and the steps of a stricturoplasty operation

Colectomy and proctocolectomy

Some patients with Crohn's affecting their large bowel (Crohn's colitis) or severely affecting the anus or rectum, may ultimately require removal of a section of the colon or sometimes the whole of the colon as well as the rectum and anus. This is called colectomy or, if rectum and anus are also removed, proctocolectomy. Medical and often alternative surgical solutions are tried before this step is taken but for a small number of Crohn's patients it is the only way to bring lasting relief from symptoms. If this operation is contemplated, your surgeon will discuss it with you in detail.

Fistulas

Fistulas occur in many people with Crohn's disease and are a common cause of surgery.

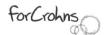

A fistula is a tunnel that runs from one surface of the body to another. Around a third to a half of all Crohn's patients experience one at some point in their lives, and the anal fistula, a tunnel between the anus and the skin of the buttock, is the most common of all. Anal fistulas are painful and leak pus. From time to time, the skin will heal over the outer end of the fistula and the pus behind will build up into a painful abscess before bursting out again.

The simplest treatment for an anal fistula is to cut it open; this usually then heals. But if the fistula is very 'high', this involves cutting through some of the muscle of the anal sphincter – leading to difficulty in controlling the bowel motions or wind – in which case, alternative operations are offered.

A seton can be placed, which is a piece of surgical thread (like cotton), passed through the fistula like an earring and then tied in a knot outside the anus. It acts as a drain and prevents the buttock hole from healing over and allows the pus to continuously drain, meaning that the cycle of abscess formation is broken. This provides great relief for many patients, but it does not heal the fistula, which continues to leak (usually a small amount of) pus.

Alternatives include the cutting seton, which cuts the fistula open slowly, allowing the sphincter to heal as the seton cuts out; advancement flaps, which involve moving a piece of skin or bowel over the fistula hole on the inside; and other advanced techniques such as fistula glue and plugs which fill the tunnel and do not involve any cutting at all. However, these techniques often fail and the main stay of treatment is now medical.

Crohn's drugs, particularly infliximab and adalimumab, have been used to heal fistulas. Nowadays, many patients will undergo surgery to control the fistula with a loose seton before getting infliximab to try and heal the fistula itself. This is probably successful in around a third of patients.

Occasionally, a stoma is used to rest the anus and encourage a fistula to heal. When all else fails and if the patient is suffering badly, the whole anus and rectum can be removed – this is called proctectomy and leads to a permanent stoma. It is rarely required for anal fistula and is seen as a last resort by surgeons and patients alike.

Always discuss the options for treatment of your fistula with both your gastroenterologist and your surgeon.

Crohn's disease from the patients

The following section looks at the accounts of six people who have undergone surgery for Crohn's disease, and offers an insight into the realities of surgery while illustrating the longer-term benefits that can be achieved. Everyone's experience of surgery is very different, so this may not necessarily be reflective of your own.

It is worth bearing in mind that people who have had a harder experience of surgery are more likely to remember it in detail and write about it, while the majority who have a much smoother experience are less likely to write about it. As such, a disproportionate number of the stories below reflect a difficult experience, and it's important to remember that you are more likely to have an operation without complications. But even those who do have difficulties, like those discussed below, describe how things have been much better for them in the long term, suggesting that even when the path is rocky, there is light at the end of the tunnel.

Cassie

After going into hospital with what was supposed to be appendicitis, Cassie was diagnosed with Crohn's. She had many difficult teenage years dominated by illness and hospital admissions, but then reached remission and was able to get her BA in film and drama, meet her future husband, buy a house, start training for her dream job as a nurse and have a gorgeous baby boy! Below, Cassie discusses her relapse and consequent surgery after the birth of her son.

"I became ill again shortly after giving birth, and months and months of drug treatment ensued. I tried everything. I was on azathioprine, Humira, Pentasa and iron tablets, and was still deteriorating. Eating was painful and opening my bowel was excruciating...worse pain than giving birth! I was off work, and for the days my son wasn't in nursery, my parents were coming to help me as I couldn't look after him properly. Not only was I tired, but I could spend up to an hour stuck on the toilet. This was my lowest point; I have a very high pain threshold, but the constant episodes on the toilet made me cry. I honestly don't know how I carried on for so

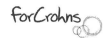

long. *A more sensible person wouldn't have!* [1] I had investigations that showed severe inflammation in my terminal colon, and it was suggested I would need a colostomy in future. The following months are a bit of a blur. I was living on soup and *Fortisip drinks* [2] as I couldn't tolerate food, and all I really remember is wondering how I was going to get out of bed each day. Having my son was a blessing because it forced me to keep going, but it also meant I couldn't rest when I needed to. A toddler is really hard work, even when you're healthy, and my little boy has been a ball of energy since the day he was born…I just couldn't keep up!

In April 2011, I was taken in for a colostomy. I was terrified. A stoma was the one thing I had never wanted. I was constantly assured that I'd pick it up easily with my healthcare background, but that wasn't the point. I wasn't worried about coping with the mechanics of it, I just did not want a stoma. I thought my husband would be appalled and never look at me the same again. I thought my son would be freaked out, and above all else, I thought I'd never be able to have more children. Despite being given plenty of opportunity, I chose not to talk about these fears. They seemed trivial, and to be honest, I was too exhausted to talk about it. That was a mistake. I'd recommend anyone in a similar situation to talk to their *stoma nurse* [3] about everything, they are amazing people and nothing embarrasses or shocks them. I talked to people who had stomas and one comment was

> **1. Phil (Surgeon) says:**
> Cassie is hard on herself but it is certainly true that patients often struggle on in a pretty awful state. Your doctors only know how bad things are if you tell them – if they don't see you or you say everything is going OK, they will assume you're OK.

> **2. Phil (Surgeon) says:**
> Fortisip drinks are dietary supplements which try to boost nutrition.

> **3. Phil (Surgeon) says:**
> Cassie is absolutely right, the stoma nurses are not just there to teach you how to use a bag, but to address any fears or problems the stoma or just the thought of one raises. They've heard it all before and have learned from other patients how to manage with problems, passing on the experience of other patients to you.

unanimous…that having a stoma had changed their lives for the better. I really wanted to feel positive about this, but just couldn't at the time.

When I came round from surgery, I was confused, as the stoma seemed to be on the wrong side. The surgeon explained that the disease was higher than they thought, and they had managed to save my rectum – so instead, he had rejoined the bowel and formed a temporary loop ileostomy to allow it to heal. I had been blocked for so long that there was a lot of old debris (aka poo) in my bowel, so they had inserted a drain to help this pass out. Unfortunately, the next day I developed an infection and had a rough week! I still felt sick and couldn't eat, so was put on *TPN* [4] for five days…again, I was stupidly resistant, scared of having a neck line inserted. It took three different doctors and a dietitian to get through to me that I needed it. I can be very stubborn! As soon as the treatment started, I knew it was the right decision because my energy returned and I was able to go for little walks around the ward. I was in for two weeks, and got home just in time for my fifth wedding anniversary.

Life with a stoma has been nothing like I imagined. I can honestly say I haven't felt so well in years. I have battled with *sore skin around the site* [5] (and still do), but it is a minor annoyance and far outweighed by the fact I can now eat! Oh yes, I can eat vegetables, fruit and all the things I have had to avoid for years! You've never seen someone smile the way I did the first time I ate a carrot. I kept wincing, waiting for the pain to start as it hit my gut, but of course it didn't happen! I have had the stoma for seven months and it is just a part of me now. In fact I'm so well that I am reticent about the reversal, and putting it off, but that's another story.

My son is not freaked out at all. He was curious for a couple of weeks, wanted to watch me change the bag and found it hysterical if any poo came out while I had it uncovered, but that interest has waned, as it does with a three year old. I am happy to say that my husband doesn't find me repulsive, as I'd imagined he would. If it bothers him at all, he hides it very well; in fact it was me who had more of a problem re-starting our sex life, as I was just so self-conscious. Nothing he said could reassure me that I wasn't hideous; I just wasn't ready to listen. All it took

4. Phil (Gastro) says:
TPN is total parenteral (bypassing the gut) nutrition. Your complete dietary requirements are delivered through a tube in the vein and when the gut is not working, usually temporarily after surgery, this allows you to receive nutrition (in the form of fat, glucose and proteins) and helps promote healing without having to wait for the gut to get going first. It helps to 'rest' the gut. A central line is often placed into the jugular vein, which is a safe procedure but a little more involved and uncomfortable than a normal cannula in your arm.

5. Phil (Surgeon) says:
This sore skin occurs because the contents of the ileostomy bag irritate the skin; the digestive enzymes in the ileum try to break down the skin it touches. Colostomies do not suffer with this problem, so the shape of the ileostomy is more of a spout to protect the skin and the bags are cut closer to the stoma too.

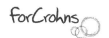

was a bit of time, and an encouraging voice in my ear by way of my fabulous sister, to realise it was me with the problem and I really did just need to open my eyes and see that everyone else was fine with it.

I have always kept my problems to myself, buried my head in the sand and tried to carry on like nothing is wrong. In some ways, this has really helped. I managed to keep working far more than people expected and have developed a strength I never knew possible. However, I'd like to urge readers not to be so stubborn. It has been my downfall at times – who knows how many months of feeling ill I'd have saved if I'd listened to my family and sought help earlier. I pushed my body to the brink, and it didn't really benefit anyone. I'd also like to encourage everyone to use the support available to them. I had access to an advice line run by the IBD nurses at my hospital, and they were wonderful. From small worries about meds or blood tests to major problems leading to me being admitted, they were always there to help. They patiently listened to me blub down the phone on my worst days, and stayed late at clinic to get my medication through when it had taken three hours to get a cannula in. I cannot praise the IBD nurses enough and I believe they deserve so much more recognition than they get.

Today I find myself smiling, because I can see a light at the end of the tunnel. I wouldn't say I was 100 per cent well; I get tired really quickly and am still dealing with the emotional turmoil of everything that has happened…but I am working full-time on a busy ward, studying to further my career and have the energy to take my son to the park, play football with him and do all the things a 30 year old should do… As long as I get into my bed by 10pm, I can take on the world, Crohn's be damned!"

Adam

Adam was diagnosed with Crohn's at the age of 11, although cannot remember a time through primary school when he was not complaining of an upset stomach. Adam has tried many options in a bid to control his Crohn's, from a range of drugs and steroids, to the meal replacement 'elemental' diet, to the more alternative medicines such as seeing a medical herbalist, a hypnotist, and an acupuncturist. After a tough journey managing life with Crohn's through his teenage years, Adam successfully joined music college and talks below about his relapse after leaving university.

"After leaving university, I had my most profound, life-altering flare-up since being diagnosed. I should preface this by explaining about my final year at uni. In my final year, I had some problems with a person I was living with, but it was a difficult situation to get out of, so it was a case of just keeping my head down and persevering. I had a lot of pent-up stress due to my living situation, and so I sought refuge in a local martial arts club. Luckily, this club was very friendly and sociable, so it provided a great outlet for some of my stress. There are two things I have always strongly believed about my relationship with Crohn's. Stress, though possibly not the cause, definitely exacerbates it. I also believe that sometimes, if you know you have a difficult period to get through, you find the strength to get through it, but then the Crohn's will often manifest itself once you have come away from the stress and 'let your guard down'. This is why I believe my next serious flare-up began a couple of months after returning home from uni.

Over the last couple of years, I have tried *tacrolimus, methotrexate, infliximab, and Humira* [6] – in that order. While all of these helped to some extent, none of them completely got me into a long period of remission. In October 2010, I eventually ended up in A&E. I remember it very clearly, as it was a Sunday morning, and I had played a gig the night before. I was so weak, so I had someone with me to dismantle my drums and pack them into my car for me. I knew something was wrong, but when you have a disease like this, you grow determined to not let it stop you living your life, so I stubbornly went ahead with the gig. I had been getting very bad fevers, lost my appetite, and was losing weight and strength. These were new symptoms to me and my Crohn's.

After not too long a wait in A&E, I was seen and immediately sent for scans of all sorts. It turned out that I had a *perianal abscess and fistula* [7]. It was surgically drained, and I was in and out of hospital three times over the month, until I eventually started to get better. To put this in context, I had been on methotrexate successfully for about ten months, and was then put on infliximab, which was stopped when I went into hospital with the abscess. At the end of this hospital stay, I was put on to Humira. This initially worked very well for me, and I was feeling really good into the New Year of January 2011.

Mid-way through January, things started to tail off again, and the Humira was clearly losing

6. Phil (Gastro) says:
These are different, very strong, immunosuppressant and 'anti-TNF' medications, discussed in more detail in the Drugs chapter.

7. Phil (Surgeon) says:
An abscess is a collection of pus and a fistula is a tunnel of infection from the inside of the anus to the skin of the buttock - they are common in Crohn's.

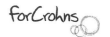

its effect. It was then that the dreaded seven-letter word was first uttered by my doctors. SURGERY. I like to think of myself as a fairly pragmatic person, who after living this long with Crohn's, has become mature enough to deal with any possible scenario in a rational manner. My heart sank! I felt that I had battled with my disease for the last ten plus years, only to be told now that I need to have surgery. Still, I eventually came to terms with it, met my surgeon, who was so nice, patient, and understanding.

I actually recorded my first consultation with him, just so that I could make sure I asked all my questions, and remember everything he said to me. I was given *two choices* [8]. The first was what they call a 'sub-total colectomy'. This involved removing a big chunk of the right side of my colon, which was the worst affected part. The hope would be that removing the area with the worst disease would allow the rest of it to heal. This would leave me with an ileostomy, with possibility of reversal. The other option was to have the whole colon and rectum removed, and to have a *permanent stoma* [9] – a 'total colectomy'. This was obviously a more drastic option, and would not leave me with many options should the disease reoccur somewhere else in the body. I decided to go for the first option. It was to be done on 1st July 2011. As it was planned surgery, I had time to seek advice from people who'd had the procedure, which I did. I came across a wonderful series of videos on YouTube, made by a girl from Newcastle in her late twenties. She made a whole video diary starting from before the surgery, right through the recovery process. This really helped me prepare myself mentally, as it gave me a good idea of what I could expect. It also prompted more questions for me to pose to my surgeon.

During the period leading up to my surgery, I continued to get weaker and was experiencing more continual pain. I was only told after the surgery that my surgeon had told my family, "Really, he's too ill to have the surgery, but he is

8. Phil (surgeon) says:

The reasons for offering these two options and the benefits of either are too complex to discuss here. When your surgeon suggests two types of operation for a given problem, ensure they give you a clear description of the advantages and disadvantages of each. Neither is likely to be 'better' per se, rather, one may suit an individual better than the other and only you, with the help of your surgeon, can decide which is best in your case.

9. Phil (surgeon) says:

Stomas are either potentially reversible or permanent and if you're offered a stoma or told one might happen it should be made very clear to you whether the intention is for a reversible or permanent stoma.

also too ill not to have it". It was early on a Friday morning, and I was first on my surgeon's list. He came to check I was ok, and then I remember seeing him briefly once I was wheeled into the anaesthetic room, all scrubbed up and ready...

As I try to recall my next memory, I am not sure when it was... I remember not being on a ward, but being on a special high-dependency unit or HDU. I remember I was in a little side room which barely had enough room to arrange some chairs around my bed. I had more tubes attached to me than I care to remember, and I remember being told to keep my little oxygen supply over my mouth. I couldn't really move. Out of my whole 'life with Crohn's' experience, this was probably my toughest time. My family were there, though I'm not sure if I managed to acknowledge them or not. I remember the first time I tried to stand up. I had lost about 20kg from my 'healthy weight'. I was so weak that the physio didn't even try to get me to take any steps at first. My next memory was on the following Monday, being moved to a side room on the ward. It was very hot, so I asked for my bed to be moved next to the window. What I was too out of it to realise was that by the time night came, it started to get really cold. Although I could move, I could not get out of bed on my own, so I was lying in the cold, waiting for a nurse to come and help me. This was a very strong emotional memory, and I remember feeling completely trapped within my own body. A lovely old Jamaican nurse, who I came to see as a grandma figure, turned up and helped me with some extra blankets. From this point on, I started to get better, albeit not quite on the *Enhanced Recovery Program* [10] they had planned for me, but I got there. Two weeks after my surgery, I was finally sent home.

I have now been living with the ileostomy for just over four months. I think under normal circumstances I would have found it very difficult to adapt to the changes that it inflicts upon one's life, but having come from such a state of desperation, I think an *equally desperate sense of determination was born, and this has seen me embrace it* [11]. I tell my friends and family about it, and people are generally quite interested. If anything, I sometimes

10. Phil (surgeon) says:
Enhanced recovery is a program designed to allow patients to recover more quickly from an operation. Adam was unlikely to make a rapid recovery given his poor nutritional state pre-op, but elements of the ER program may still help avoid complications and speed up recovery.

11. Lucy (IBD Nurse):
It can be very emotional and stressful having to have surgery and a stoma. IBD Nurses can support you through this difficult time and help you adjust to your new life.

80

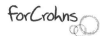

have to be careful not to explain some things too explicitly. I am feeling very well, and back to a relatively normal working life – well, as normal as a working life can be for a freelance musician!"

Sally

Sally is a 28-year-old woman who has had Crohn's disease for five years. She tells us about the difficult times she went through upon finding out she needed an ileostomy. She also talks about the process of recovery and moving forward after her surgery.

"Before I tell you my story, I want to tell you that there is a happy ending. Unfortunately, reading about surgery is never going to be all sweetness and light, and I don't want to sugar-coat anything, but I want you to know that I truly believe that surgery can improve your life – and more importantly – it can save your life. Please don't be scared of anything that I talk about. Everyone's experience with Crohn's disease is so different and mine has not been an easy journey. However, as you will read, it can also have a really positive impact on your life. It has made me appreciate small things so much more; it has made me a more caring and understanding person, and has ignited my fighting spirit! So here's my story…

"The only option is an ileostomy". As soon as I heard those words, for the second time in my life, I screamed. Not just a slight scream, but a rather loud and bellowing, blood-curdling scream. The age-old question, 'why me?' pops into your head. 'What have I done to deserve this?' The problem with Crohn's is that no one can even tell me how I got it. Every day I wonder if I did something wrong, if I ate too many cheeseburgers, or don't eat enough foods with vitamin C or D. Maybe *I did something* [12] really bad in a previous life, which means I am being punished this time around. I still drive myself mad on a daily basis, desperately searching for answers, but no one can tell me how or why I have it, I just do.

> **12. Phil (Gastro) says:**
> Sally did nothing to cause her Crohn's disease. The cause is not fully understood but there is a strong genetic component which leads to a malfunctioning immune defence system. More details on the cause of Crohn's can be found in section 1.

After recently recovering from a reversal operation after five months of unbelievable pain, here I am again. What a waste of five months of my life. I was surprised to hear that the Crohn's hadn't reappeared when they joined me up, which is fairly common; instead it was attacking my rectum. An *ileostomy* [13], or be incontinent for the rest of my life. Not a normal decision for a 24 year old to make, when most of my friends are trying to decide which new nightclub to go to, or which new dress to buy. Obviously ileostomy won over being incontinent, but to this day, that was the most depressing night of my life. As I lay in that hospital bed, staring out of the window over a fantastic view of London, I didn't stop stroking my already scarred stomach, almost saying goodbye to it – saying goodbye to normality. People say that it is like losing a limb. It sounds silly, but it is. Most 24 year olds are worried if their tummy looks flat enough for a bikini on their summer holiday. I, meanwhile, have to try and conjure up ingenious ways to cover mine, not because I'm fat, but because hidden away, under my cleverly-constructed outfits is a bag full of waste. Delightful, eh?

Let me start at the beginning. When I was first diagnosed with Crohn's, I was relieved; relieved to finally have a name for the pain and suffering that had invaded my life for the past eight months. I thought I'd take a few tablets and be able to get my life back. No such luck. Doctors have since told me I have an incredibly aggressive form of Crohn's. In a matter of months it had developed so badly that I was bed ridden, ulcers covering my whole digestive system, including my gullet. I couldn't even swallow water without wincing. Going to the loo 28+ times a day. I can tell you all the ingredients of every item in my bathroom, as I would get so bored sat on the loo, I would read literally anything! Eventually, after my second hospitalisation, a scan to check whether my NG food tube was inserted properly showed two *perforations* [14] in my bowel. Not something you want to hear. Being operated on at midnight is scary. You know quite how serious it is. I was so weak and on so many painkillers that I couldn't quite get my head around the enormity of what was about to take place. My surgeon assured me that if they could fix me

13. Phil (Surgeon) says:
When a temporary stoma is placed, to protect a surgical join and decrease the risk of a leak, that stoma can be 'reversed', meaning the bowel is joined again at the stoma site and the waste goes back to its normal route out via the anus. It is usually a more minor operation than the original when the stoma was created.

14. Phil (Surgeon) says:
Perforations are holes in the wall of the bowel that let the waste and enzymes from your gut leak into the rest of the body. This is called peritonitis and is very dangerous indeed. It is not common but an operation is urgently needed as in Sally's case.

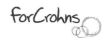

up without an ileostomy, they would, but alas they couldn't. Coming round from an operation is always a blur. You don't tend to care about anything in the world because you're on so many drugs. It took me a few days of being in intensive care to realise that I had nearly lost my life. That the Crohn's diagnosis I was originally so glad to hear was in fact not as simple as I'd first thought. As I lay in bed with people beeping on life support machines around me, I felt grateful that I was alive and keen to pick myself up and get on with things as quickly as possible.

Lying in intensive care, attached to millions of beeping wires (including lines coming out of my neck) *made it hard to keep positive* [15]. My first aim was to be able to lift my arms. From being so malnourished, I had oedema, which is albumin build-up in my limbs. It looked like someone had quite literally inflated me. My arms and legs were at bursting point. As days went on, I could eventually lift my heavy arms and the albumin started to disappear.

No one warns you about situations like this, rare as it is. We often all assume that Crohn's is just

> **15. Phil (Surgeon) says:**
> This must have been a scary moment. The lines are fine plastic tubes which can be placed into veins and arteries for monitoring and giving drugs and fluids. Other tubes are sometimes placed into the bladder or stomach during an operation and are removed soon afterwards.

restricted to your digestive system, but it's not. After a week of physio, I managed to swing my legs off the bed, a huge achievement. Standing up was still too hard. There was too much weight, and I was too scared. Every day the physio would come back, until eventually I managed to stand with a zimmer.

By this time the albumin had gone, and I was on a normal ward, no longer in intensive care. I managed to walk to the bathroom with encouraging smiles and cheers from patients around me. I'll never forget looking at myself in the mirror for the first time in weeks. The colour had gone from my face, my hair was thinning and my ordinary curvy size 10-12 figure had disappeared to a scrawny, child-like frame. Bones were sticking out where they shouldn't, my boobs had disappeared, and it was a scared little girl staring back at me. At this point, I was hoping that the stretch marks that encased my legs would fade over time. Five years later, they are still there, a constant reminder of those dark times, when I was unable to walk. This was to be another obstacle to overcome when choosing what to wear. No bare legs for me in summer. I get people asking what's wrong with my legs, or people just staring at them.

After months and months of recovery, and vast amounts of food and protein shakes, I began to piece my life back together. How do you though? Everything feels like it's been turned upside down. The final obstacle I had to overcome was losing my hair. The stress of surgery and the strong medications I was on meant it pretty much all fell out. No one can prepare you for how that makes you feel. Already hating the scrawny child-like image of myself in the mirror, with an ileostomy and now also balding! My mum took me wig shopping, and after finding one that didn't look too dissimilar from my own hair (apart from being a lot more styled and pristine!) I felt a little better, apart from the headaches you get from wearing a wig all day. Over the next few weeks, I started becoming more and more independent, and eventually went back to work part-time, and then a month later full-time. I think it was at this point that it suddenly dawned on me what a huge ordeal I had been through. When you are ill, you are focusing on getting better and better each day, but once you resume normal activity, it suddenly feels very strange. I spent the next year and a half concentrating solely on being able to have a reversal; when they eventually gave me a date and told me it could go ahead I was ecstatic. The date I needed to go into hospital was a Sunday in June 2008, the same day as Walk forCrohn's. I decided to go along with my two best friends, my boyfriend and my mum. It was a very emotional experience, as all I could keep thinking was 'in a few hours I'm going to be in hospital, and the next day I'm going to have the reversal'. I was so excited that I'd forgotten there was going to be a long road to recovery after the operation.

I remember waking up in the recovery room after my reversal, completely out of it, but all I could think was 'is it gone?' I asked the nurse, who told me 'yes, it has all gone to plan'. That meant I could sleep easily, knowing my life would be back to normal. It took me weeks and weeks to recover, it was hard work. I'd forgotten what it was like to spend so much time on the loo, the trusty stack of trashy mags was back in the bathroom! It hurt every time I went, and I used to sit on the loo and sob, but I was strangely happy that I was able to go to the toilet like a 'normal person'. In some sick way, the pain was almost satisfying. I was so excited about being able to wear low-slung jeans, tight-fitting tops and slinky dresses. I often walked around the house with my top rolled up, happy to expose my scarred belly, happy to be able to show it off again, happy to be able to rub it. I was proud of those scars, proud to be able to expose them.

After a few months, I went back to work; it was hard. I needed to go to the loo quite a lot, and it didn't feel quite right. Then I started to get very weak, I had to take time off work and spend most of my days on the loo, blood and mucus pouring out of me, with no real control. This was scary. I was taken straight to hospital to see my consultant. By this point, I was so weak and in so much pain that I needed a wheelchair. It wasn't good news. My consultant found me a bed in the hospital straight away, ordered tests, and when the surgeon came in a few days later, he told me I had one of the most diseased rectums he had seen in a long time. It was

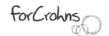

so bad that he took a picture on his iPhone; I declined the offer to look at it! That was it, there was no choice but to give it time to rest, time to heal and to give me back the ileostomy. With the screams that came out of my mouth, you would've thought I'd just been given a death sentence! Nothing could console me; I was devastated. Nothing and no one could calm me down. Three days later I had the operation. I remember the morning before, stroking my tummy, sobbing, staring at it in the mirror, saying goodbye to it. Who knew if I would ever see it again without the ileostomy bag on it? I felt so frustrated that I had spent months recovering from the reversal, just for my body to let me down, and for the Crohn's to develop in a completely new place. My intestines were in perfect order, no Crohn's at all. It had decided to attack me in the rectum. It just didn't seem fair.

The months recovering from my third operation were really hard. It was an operation I really didn't want. It was coming up to Christmas, I was weak, tired and exhausted with life; but I knew I had to pick myself up and carry on. I had coped with it before and I would cope with it again. This was not going to beat me.

Almost four years on from my third operation, I am still with the ileostomy. It's not ideal, but when I think about the hours spent sobbing on the loo, in such pain, I question why I would want to go back to that again. I manage to work full-time, I manage to go out with my friends, go on holiday, wear normal clothes and do pretty much anything that I want to. I am so lucky I have such fantastic people around me, who make me want to get up every day and fight the Crohn's. I've decided to have a reversal in the next few months, but it isn't a decision I've taken lightly. I have had to consider if it is worth the risk and the trauma of the operation. Ultimately I have decided I need to give it one more go. I'm fully prepared, emotionally, for it to fail again, but I'm going into it with a positive outlook and I'm hopeful that it will work. I will beat this hideous disease and have my tummy back again.

Having an ileostomy doesn't change you as a person. Plenty of people know I have it, and plenty of people don't. I don't find it necessary to tell everyone I meet that I have one, mainly because I don't want to be treated differently, but I don't think it's something to be ashamed of. Without it, I'd be dead. The perforated bowel would've made sure of that! I had to have it the second time or let my rectum become more diseased and be permanently incontinent. I think that would've been an even worse choice. My main desire now is to lead a happy, healthy, normal life and hopefully get married one day and start a family – with or without the ileostomy. Being alive is the most important thing to me, and being able to lead as normal a life as I possibly can, never letting the Crohn's beat me."

Sue

Sue is 59 and has had Crohn's disease for over 30 years. She talks of her operation to remove a blockage and her positive experiences since.

"I had an operation many years ago to remove a blockage. The operation was planned, and I had to be on fluids for about six weeks before having the operation. At the time, I actually welcomed the surgery as I had a great deal of faith in my surgeon.

The operation certainly improved my health. Before surgery, I was in pain, lost weight, passed out and did not pass motion. After the surgery, the pain stopped immediately. It did take me time to get over the operation however, because I had problems with the nasal tube and couldn't pass urine, so I had a catheter that stayed in for some time. I would have liked to have been *told in advance* [16] about the tubes that I had to have.

I was in hospital for approximately three and a half weeks, but as the operation was in 1976, I am sure the techniques have changed greatly now. I understand that they can now do the operation by *keyhole, and therefore one would only be in hospital for just day* [17].

Now I have put on weight (too much!) and am no longer in pain. I am, however, back on medication as the area operated on has narrowed and I still have frequent visits to the toilet. Despite all this, I have always led a very normal and busy life, and will continue to do so.

My family and friends gave me tremendous support and I returned to work six weeks after the operation, and continuing my hectic work schedule. Apart from one comment blurted out by an idiot about my operation scar, while on holiday, I have never had any other comments, and really have always led a normal life."

16. Phil (surgeon) says:
This is usually explained to patients, but if you have any questions when an operation is planned, then write them down and ask your surgeon or their team when you see them.

17. Phil (surgeon) says:
Sue is right when she says that keyhole operations can speed up recovery and get patients back on their feet quicker.

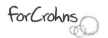

Kelsea

Kelsea is 22 years old and training to be a midwife. She shares her experiences of having fistulas and the resulting surgery and after care.

"From April 2011 to the present day, I have had seven operations, six of these for fistula-related issues. I'd just had a successful *hemi-colectomy* [18] operation and was at home recovering when I suddenly felt a strange pain around my *perineum* [19], which also sent pains down my leg. The GP said it could be a trapped nerve, however I was convinced it was an abscess. A couple of days after seeing my GP, I was rushed to hospital in excruciating pain, taken to surgery where they discovered a relatively deep *abscess* [20], which was subsequently drained.

Being rather naïve to perianal Crohn's disease, I thought once it had healed that would be it. This was however not the case. I developed another abscess, and after having *an MRI scan* [21], they discovered that I had a fistula. This meant going for day surgery and having seton stitches placed.

Honestly, I had no idea what these were, and after doing some research, I was not looking forward to it. The thought of having loops of material running through the fistulas and out of my anus was terrifying! However I knew this had to be done to stop the pain, so I had the surgery.

18. Phil (surgeon) says:
Hemi-colectomy: This is removal of part of the bowel which is discussed more above – what happened next is not specifically related to the operation and you shouldn't worry that the one will lead to the other.

19. Phil (surgeon) says:
Perineum: This is the sensitive area of skin between the vagina or scrotum and the anus itself.

20. Phil (surgeon) says:
Abscesses in this area can be terribly painful although that pain gets much better very quickly after the abscess is 'drained' which means taking the top off like a boiled egg so the pus inside can drain out.

21. Phil (surgeon) says:
This is the best way to see the extent of a fistula using imaging. Ultrasound scans are also used and examination under general anaesthetic (EUA) is often the most useful way to assess a fistula.

I had draining setons inserted [22]. These do not cut through the fistula like the "cutting" setons do, they just stay in place to keep the fistula open to allow for the pus to drain. Everyone reacts differently to these operations. My first operation was a shock to say the least; I looked in the mirror at my bottom end and burst into tears, I had massive wounds, one larger than a 50p piece and so very deep!

After the initial shock of how it looked, I began to think about how I would live a normal life. How would I maintain a relationship with my partner? How would I go to the toilet? How could I do the basic things that many take for granted? There was also the thought of aftercare, which is crucial after this type of surgery.

I had four more operations after this, to add more stitches (after finding new branches to a fistula) and to drain a labial abscess which also links to my fistulas.

By now, I am a pro at looking after my fistulas! Having lots of hot baths helps to soothe any initial pain, which usually passes after a couple of weeks. While in the hot bath, I *move my stitches* [23] to keep the holes as wide as possible, to allow the pus to drain easily. Flushing the wounds with a saline solution also helps me and removes pus. I wear pads and dressings at all times as the setons constantly drain pus, and initially sat on a ring to ease the pain. I use a shower to clean myself after using the toilet to avoid irritating my stitches and damaging my skin.

I found that doctors and surgeons do the surgery, give you some information and send you on your way. For this reason, my main piece of advice for anyone having surgery for fistulas is to get in touch with your IBD nurse. My IBD nurse is a life-saver, I still see her regularly now and she gives my fistulas a good flush.

22. Phil (surgeon) says:
This is a good example of when you need to know what's going to be done before you go into theatre. One type of seton is there to try to heal the fistula, the other simply prevents further abscess but remains there and leads to ongoing drainage. Talk to your surgeon so you know what you're having done and what it will achieve.

23. Phil (surgeon) says:
This is important. Kelsea knows what her operation was for. The knot of the seton can sometimes get stuck in the outer hole of the fistula and block the drainage – an abscess can then appear. She is making sure that she has the best chance of avoiding future problems.

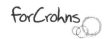

She was the one who provided me with the most information about looking after my setons. Another piece of advice is not to be afraid. I am not going to say it doesn't change your life, because it does, but like any other issue that comes with Crohn's, *you learn to adapt. Never feel alone!"* [24]

> **24. Lucy (IBD Nurse):**
> IBD nurses are very experienced dealing with these types of problems and are happy to be contacted at any time about such issues.

Summary

When a patient has to undergo surgery, they and their families are inevitably worried, even frightened, unsure and feel out of control. As you've seen, although surgery is a daunting prospect, it can make an enormous and positive difference, giving a long period of remission from symptoms and improving your quality of life. Conversations with the surgeon to understand the operation have really helped several of the authors, and an open and honest discussion about what to expect, how recovery is likely to go, what risks exist, and so on, is very valuable. Most people worry that they will end up with a stoma for the rest of their lives. These are usually not necessary, but when they are, it is for safety – to reduce the risks of the operation, improve your outcome, and they are usually temporary. Your surgeon will tell you whether one is likely and whether it is temporary. The reality of a stoma is always better than the fears patients have pre-op. It's worth remembering that no one will know you have one unless you want them to – you'll almost certainly have met someone with a stoma in the last few months, you just didn't know it.

Tips and suggestions

The following tips and suggestions are taken from the authors of our stories and healthcare professionals about their experiences of surgery.

- **Ask for an explanation**
  If you don't understand something, it's usually because it hasn't been adequately explained. Doctors will assume you understand something if you don't question it. You will be able to deal with anything that happens much better if you know what it means, and most doctors will be happy to give you all the information you want for this reason.

- **Be patient**
  Expect things to take longer than you'd like.
  If you think things are taking too long, then ask your nurse or doctor, but generally all departments are busy and prioritise according to clinical need, so waiting longer for something is usually good news.

- **Discuss alternatives**
  If you've heard of a different way to do something then bring it up. Your doctor will not assume you're questioning their competence or the decision they've made, and like patients to be actively involved in their own care. There is usually a straight-forward answer as to why one option is better than another in any given situation.

- **Food and fluids are important**
  You can ask for a supplementary menu which is higher in calories and easier to digest – your ward dietician can help with this.
  If you are a fussy eater, make sure you eat something (if you are allowed to). Hospital food isn't always the best, but you need to build your strength back up! Ask a family member or friend to bring you in suitable alternatives (although it may not be possible to warm this up on the wards). This does not mean that you should be eating junk food though! Have a constant supply of bottled water by your bed.

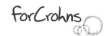
- **Take comfy pyjamas (or ideally nightdresses if you're a girl**
  You may be in hospital gowns for days but it's always so much nicer when you can change into your own clothes. All of these small things begin to make you feel more human again. Choose something that either has a huge elasticated waistline or a nightdress if you're a girl.

- **If you're tired, tell people**
  If you are tired, get in touch with a friend or family member and tell them that you are not feeling up to visitors that day. Sometimes it can be exhausting when you just want to sleep and you have lots of people who want to chat. Don't feel that you need to talk for hours on the phone, or have visitors constantly. Remember you are in hospital to rest!

- **Don't push yourself too hard, but do push yourself**
  If you are told you need to walk around the ward four times a day - DO IT! But if one day you are feeling too weak and dizzy, speak to the nurse or your consultant first. Don't do it if you know you are going to faint, that's going to set you back. Use your common sense. Sometimes things are going to be a little painful and uncomfortable, but you still need to do it if the physio or doctor has told you to. Set yourself little goals and try and reach them, you will feel better for it.

- **Expect bad days after surgery**
  People often feel good the first day after surgery, but a day or two later, they feel as if they're going backwards. This is very common and does not usually mean something has gone wrong. Your doctor will take a careful look at you if you feel worse one day, but these backward steps are generally short-lived and happen to many people. The key is not to panic and to know that two steps forward, one step back is quite a common way to progress.

- **Don't pack everything you own**
  You're in hospital because you are ill, so keep it simple – don't pack a 20kg suitcase (you have very little storage space in hospital). It can become frustrating if you can't do all of the activities you bring

along with you, but most of the time, you probably won't have the concentration or energy to do much except rest. If you do begin to feel better, your friends and family can bring more things in for you, and as soon as you are well enough, you'll be at home watching DVDs and playing games to your heart's content.

Take a good book or two, and some money for the hospital TV, but don't bother buying magazines (family and friends will buy millions for you).

Tips and suggestions - fistulas

The following tips and suggestions are taken from those with Crohn's and healthcare professionals about their experiences of how to care for fistulas.

- **Speak to your Stoma/ IBD nurses**
  Stoma/IBD nurses can offer great support and information on how to care for your fistulas.

- **Take lots of hot baths**
  Take lots of hot baths to help soothe any initial pain.

- **Move your stitches**
  The knot of the seton can sometimes get stuck in the outer hole of the first fistula and block the drainage, which can cause an abscess.
  While in a hot bath, move your stitches to keep the holes as wide as possible – this allows the pus to drain easily.

- **Flush your wounds**
  Flushing your wounds with a saline solution can help soothe and remove any pus

- **Use a shower after going to the toilet**
  Use a shower to clean yourself after using the toilet to avoid irritating stitches and damaging your skin.

- **Dress the wound**
  Wear pads and dressing at all times, as the setons constantly drain pus.

Nutrition and diet in Crohn's disease

Diet and nutrition are a big part of anyone's life, but it is particularly important for those with Crohn's disease to understand how it can affect them. This chapter explains the different types of nutritional advice and treatment, which can help patients with Crohn's.

Crohn's disease from the medics

Patients with Crohn's can often feel out of control or that their condition is taking over their life. Changing your diet to ensure that it is as balanced as possible can help patients feel like they are positively contributing to their health – minimising the risk of malnutrition and helping the immune system deal with inflammation caused by Crohn's.

Can diet cause Crohn's disease?

When first diagnosed with Crohn's disease, many patients ask if it is because of something they ate or as a consequence of their diet. Although research has tried to answer this question, it has not yet been possible to prove that Crohn's disease results from diet. The western diet is often implicated as a cause of Crohn's. It has been found that patients who immigrate to the west, especially those from the Indian sub-continent (changing their diet accordingly), are now developing Crohn's disease. A possible reason for this is different fats, as the western diet contains fats that are more likely to result in inflammation than other fats thought to be anti-inflammatory. This is a very difficult issue and is far from fully understood. As the development of Crohn's disease is thought to have many different risk factors, it will require much more research to answer this question.

Nutritional problems associated with Crohn's

As any part of the gastrointestinal tract can be affected by Crohn's disease, it is easy to understand how eating and drinking can become problematic. Therefore, it is really important that patients get advice from a dietitian who has a good knowledge of Crohn's disease and its consequences. The dietitian can then provide individualised advice, depending on the site of the Crohn's disease and the symptoms experienced. Everyone with Crohn's disease is different. You may know someone with Crohn's disease who has been advised to follow a particular diet, but this advice may not be suitable for you.

Patients with Crohn's can become malnourished very quickly for several reasons:

- Reduced appetite causing a reduction in food intake

- An increase in nutritional requirements resulting from Crohn's

- Side-effects of the treatments, such as nausea and vomiting

- Malabsorption due to on-going inflammation

All patients should have their Body Mass Index (BMI) calculated upon diagnosis, to act as a baseline in order to monitor changes in nutritional status and to identify those who are at risk of malnutrition. All patients in hospital should have a nutritional screening assessment completed, which will identify those at risk or already experiencing malnutrition. A common screening tool is called the Malnutrition Universal Screening Tool or MUST.

The MUST tool incorporates BMI, percentage of weight loss and an acute disease effect score, which is based on an assessment of how ill the patient is and if there has been or is likely to be no nutritional intake for more than five days. BMI is calculated as below:

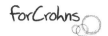

$$\text{Body mass index (BMI)} = \frac{\text{weight (kg)}}{\text{height (m) X height (m)}}$$

A MUST score of 2 or more should prompt a referral to the dietitian, as this means you are already malnourished or at high risk of becoming malnourished.

In children, this issue is of particular importance as malnutrition can affect growth. It is therefore essential that all children diagnosed with Crohn's are referred to a specialist paediatric dietitian who can provide specialist advice to minimise the effect of Crohn's on growth and development.

Furthermore, Crohn's can cause micronutrient deficiencies as discussed below.

Anaemia

Anaemia is common in patients with Crohn's and results in tiredness, which affects quality of life. Anaemia may be due to iron, folate or vitamin B12 deficiency, or a combination of the three and often arises when children are malnourished. Vitamin B12 deficiency can occur if you've had the part of your gut joining the small and large bowel (terminal ileum) removed. A regular check of your blood should highlight any deficiencies that can be treated with suitable medication and targeted diet therapy.

Osteoporosis

Osteoporosis is also common in Crohn's and has been associated with poor calcium and Vitamin D intake. Treatment with steroids is also known to increase your chances of developing osteoporosis. An assessment of your diet can highlight inadequate amounts of calcium and vitamin D, and a dietitian can provide advice on how to increase the amount of these nutrients in the diet as well as recommend suitable supplements.

Nutrition as treatment

Nutrition during active disease

The dietary management of active Crohn's focuses on three aspects of the disease:

- Achieving remission

- Reduction in symptoms

- Maintaining or improving nutritional status

One approach to the treatment of active disease is the use of a liquid diet, known as exclusive enteral nutrition. This is when patients do not eat or drink anything except specially-formulated liquids that contain all of the essential nutrients required for good health. These liquids are known as oral nutritional supplements (e.g. Ensure Plus, Fortisip, Fresubin energy drink, Modulen, Peptamen, Elemental 028). This treatment is usually required for up to eight weeks to achieve remission. After 10 days, patients should notice a difference in the symptoms, but it can take up to eight weeks to show that the lining of the gut has healed (known as mucosal healing.)

There are three different types of enteral nutrition used in Crohn's:

- Elemental: this is when the nutrition has been fully broken down into amino acids, which are the building blocks of protein.

- Semi-elemental: this is when the nutrition has been partially broken down into peptides, which are a few amino acids joined together, but still smaller than proteins.

- Polymeric: this is where the nutrition has not been broken down at all.

The choice of enteral nutrition is often based on the expertise of the team looking after people with Crohn's. Research studies comparing these different types of liquid diet have shown no difference in achieving remission, and therefore the most important factor is patient preference. It is really important that patients get to taste all the different types, as good compliance is needed in order to get the best possible results from these liquid diets. One of the most difficult aspects

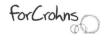

of following this diet is the lack of any other food allowed. Therefore, it is important that friends, family and the whole team looking after the person following the diet, are really supportive and readily available to give encouragement and advice when difficult circumstances arise. Some of the side-effects from these diets can be quite surprising, although often harmless (your poo may turn green), so it is vital that you are in regular contact with your dietitian to discuss these issues. You should never feel silly asking questions, as all questions are important and usually have an explanation which can help put you at ease.

Sometimes patients find it difficult to drink the volume of liquid diet recommended by the dietitian, and in this situation the diet can be given through a tube that is passed via the nose into the stomach, known as a nasogastric tube. The advantage of this tube is that the nutrition can be infused slowly during the day and the night, which can ensure that the full amount is being delivered. Some patients choose to pass their own nasogastric tube each night so that they can remove it during the day.

It is frustrating that after several decades of research, we still do not really know why these diets work. Some researchers think that it could be due to the removal of food or "bowel rest", changes in the bugs (microorganisms such as bacteria) in the gut or an effect on the immune system resulting from changes in the type of fats provided by enteral nutrition.

All patients should be offered this treatment option during active disease, but especially children, adolescents, pregnant and lactating women, or patients experiencing unpleasant side-effects from Crohn's medications.

These oral nutritional supplements can also be used to improve nutrition status in addition to usual food. It is especially important to treat malnutrition before an operation, as those who are malnourished are more likely to experience complications from surgery if their nutritional status has not been optimised.

Nutrition during remission

Once patients have completed the recommended period of time on the liquid diet, food will be reintroduced. After such a long time without any normal food, it is tempting for patients to eat everything and anything. However, it is a good idea to introduce foods back into your diet in a slow way so that your bowel can get used to dealing with solid food again. It is also important to assess if any particular foods cause symptoms and if remission can be maintained.

There has been some research about the best way to reintroduce food after a liquid diet, and you should discuss all the options with your dietitian.

The elimination diet

This involves reintroducing one food each day and assessing for effect. If a food is found to cause symptoms then it would be excluded. Research has shown that this process can be better than steroids at keeping patients in remission, but it can be time-consuming.

The LOFFLEX diet

This diet uses a similar approach as the elimination diet, but is easier and not as time-consuming and was found to result in the same level of remission. It reintroduces foods that are low in fat and fibre for 2-4 weeks, after which, other foods known to cause problems in Crohn's in some people are reintroduced one at a time and assessed for symptoms.

Once again, the choice of reintroduction is based on local expertise and patient preference. Additionally, a lot of support and encouragement is required during this process in order that the diet is followed correctly. Any foods that provoke symptoms are removed from the diet and suitable alternatives are discussed to ensure the final diet is balanced and contains the correct amount of nutrients to prevent deficiencies and malnutrition occurring. One of the most important aspects of this process is that patients are not unnecessarily excluding foods that they are not intolerant to. Research has shown that this can occur due to the nature of Crohn's, and often patients consume very restricted diets which may be unbalanced and lacking essential nutrients. Therefore a dietitian can often help in assessing symptoms during the reintroduction period, and support patients to re-try foods initially thought to cause symptoms, as often this could have occurred by coincidence.

Lactose intolerance

Many patients with Crohn's avoid milk and dairy products as they feel they result in gastrointestinal symptoms. It is known that levels of the enzyme lactase, which is responsible for breaking down lactose, reduce after intestinal resection resulting in lactose intolerance, but this is usually temporary and improves after time. The exclusion of milk and lactose-based foods can put patients at risk of osteoporosis, as they are high in calcium content. Therefore, if patients exclude lactose from their diet, a dietitian can help to ensure that suitable alternatives are suggested, and that intake of the recommended amount of calcium is achieved from food or supplements.

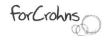

The dietary management of strictures

In Crohn's there are two types of strictures that can develop. A stricture can result from scar tissue where the bowel has recovered from inflammation, or from on-going inflammation caused by active Crohn's. The type of diet that can be managed by the patient will depend on how easy it is for food and fluid to pass through the stricture. Some people will only be able to manage liquids, as solid food can get stuck, causing pain, bloating and vomiting. Others will be able to manage some normal diet but will be advised to follow a low-fibre diet. Fibre is the part of food that does not get digested by the bowel and can therefore cause a blockage. Once again, it is important to discuss this diet with a dietitian who can advise on a suitable consistency and amount of fibre to take. They'll also assess the diet to check it is balanced and contains the correct amount of nutrients to prevent deficiencies and malnutrition occurring.

Foods that are high in fibre include fruit and vegetables (especially the skins, stalks, pips, peel and seeds), wholemeal bread, brown rice and pasta, high-fibre breakfast cereals, nuts and seeds,

Functional symptoms

It is now well known that patients with Crohn's, as well as the rest of the population, can experience gastrointestinal symptoms such as bloating, diarrhoea, pain and excessive gas production, not necessarily related to their underlying Crohn's. These symptoms may be helped by altering the type and amount of fibre in the diet. In addition, a new approach to symptom relief is the FODMAP diet. This diet aims to reduce foods that are known to ferment in the bowel, causing these symptoms and can be discussed with a dietitian.

Pre and probiotics

There has been a lot of interest in the use of pre and probiotics to improve gut health over the past decade, with several products now widely available. At present, the research conducted has not conclusively shown that the use of these products helps achieve and maintain remission, but further research continues.

Fish oil supplements

There has been a lot of research investigating the use of fish oils in several conditions resulting from inflammation. Fish oils contain two types of fat (known as

EPA and DHA) that are thought to have anti-inflammation activity. Two studies have looked at remission rates after taking fish oils, with one showing an improvement in remission and the other showing no improvement. Therefore at the moment, more research needs to be done in this area.

Summary

Lots of patients have identified that food and nutrition are a really important part of their experience of Crohn's, and many have experienced difficulties with eating. Sadly, many patients are not seen by a dietitian, so don't receive the individual assessment and advice that is desired. Patients have also requested better written information regarding their diet and nutrition, which can be provided if a referral to a dietitian is made.

Fast facts

- Crohn's can cause malnutrition and micronutrient deficiencies

- Ask for a referral to a dietitian who will give you tailored individual advice

- Don't be afraid to ask your consultant about dietary treatments

- Nutrition can be used alone or in combination with other medical treatment

- There is currently no evidence for the use of pre or probiotics in Crohn's

- More research is needed in this area

Crohn's disease from the patients

The following section looks at the experiences of six people who have used different nutritional strategies for managing their Crohn's disease. Sometimes nutrition is used as a treatment (like a drug or operation) but also the day-to-day impact of food is important in Crohn's. These stories help to illustrate both aspects.

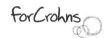

Kelsea

Kelsea is 22 and works as a student midwife. She has had Crohn's for two years and would describe it as 'moderate' in severity. Here she discusses her experience of Modulen.

"Before my Laparoscopic Right Hemicolectomy, my bowel was so ulcerated and I had a terrible stricture, so was struggling to keep any food down. My gastroenterologist and dietitian decided that I should be put on a Modulen diet for eight weeks, up until the date of my surgery. This was a shock as I did not know what this was, or how I would manage to maintain this diet. After a lot of sessions with my dietitian, I decided I would go on the Modulen diet [1]. Modulen is a liquid feed filled with all the nutrition needed by an individual. It is proven to help reduce inflammation caused by Crohn's disease. Modulen is a very strict diet; it is in powdered form which you mix with water and can add flavouring (either the one given with the Modulen or Nesquik powder). This and water is all that is allowed while being on this diet. This meant no other food, not even squashes or a cup of tea!

> **1. Phil (Gastro):**
> In children, adolescents and young adults nutrition is often used as a 'first line' treatment showing better results and outcomes than steroids.

Needless to say, I was apprehensive. I was concerned that I would not be able to follow such a strict diet for the eight weeks needed. The night before starting Modulen, I treated myself to a junk food binge (I do not recommend it for us Crohnies, but I felt I needed to do it before starting the

> **2. Alison (dietitian) says:**
> Planning and preparation is the key to any diet but this is especially true when following a difficult diet like this one.

Modulen!) and prepared myself to start. As I was working at this point, I had to work out how I would manage my diet at work and in public. I had to drink a Modulen drink every two hours during the day, all of specific measurements. This meant buying a flask to keep the drink cold, preparing all my drinks in the morning if I was going to work, and carrying lots of straws (these make it easier to drink slower, keeping you fuller for *longer*! [2])

It was a difficult period of time for me. The first two weeks were the hardest. It was hard to think of anything else other than food (or lack of) and it was difficult to adjust to the taste. After the first two weeks, it began to get easier. I started to actually enjoy the taste of Modulen (when mixed with banana flavouring, I couldn't stomach the other flavours) and I settled into the two-hourly routine. I felt better almost instantly and worked more than I had in the months previously.

Once I came off the Modulen, I went straight in for my operation. My dietitian had put a strict diet routine in place for after my surgery, as not only had I gone through serious bowel surgery, but I had not eaten solid foods for two months. I followed this as much as I could (which was difficult, as I was in hospital over Easter and came home to tonnes of Easter eggs!) and as far as my bowel problems go, I have never felt better. I still have flare-ups, but rarely, and they do not last as long as before starting Modulen. I would recommend Modulen to any person with Crohn's disease who

> **3. Alison (dietitian) says:**
> I agree that getting support in the first two weeks is essential. This is usually when the urge to eat normal food can be the worst, especially if you haven't started reaping the benefits of the diet in terms of improvement in symptoms.

has been offered it, as it really helped me, *and if you can get past the first two week hurdle, you will be fine!"* [3]

Olivia

Olivia is 17 and currently at school studying for A Levels. She was diagnosed with Crohn's when she was 10 and has had one operation. She currently describes her Crohn's as 'mild'. Here she discusses her experience of Modulen.

"I was 10 years old when I first experienced symptoms of severe fatigue, stomach pains and weight loss. After lots of prodding and poking from various doctors, as well as a blood test, barium test, MRI scan, colonoscopy and endoscopy, I was diagnosed with Crohn's disease in 2005. Being so young at the time, I found it difficult to understand the illness in more detail than 'my white blood cells attacking my insides', I know now to be part of my ileum. Shortly after this, I was put on the Modulen diet to allow the damaged part of my small intestine to calm down – it had become highly inflamed and scarred.

The diet consisted of drinking 2400ml of Modulen a day, which I broke up into eight 300ml cups. As I was strictly banned from eating or drinking anything else during the eight-week diet, I tried to keep a structure to my day. I did this

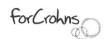

by having a cup for breakfast, a cup at break time, two cups at lunch, a cup after school, two cups for dinner and a last cup before *bed* [4]. Modulen contains all the nutrients a person could need, so amazingly I never found myself feeling hungry. Of course, the full-up feeling never stopped me from craving crisps and chocolate, but not giving in to these desires allowed me to develop a strong power of self-discipline and determination.

There is no doubt that an eight-week diet like this can strongly affect one's lifestyle – not being able to eat out at parties or restaurants. It's also true that Crohn's disease does affect your social life, especially as a teenager, because it's difficult to make friends when you're constantly missing school – trust me. But I do strongly believe that the effect it can have is all down to how much you let it affect you. I tried to find fun ways to get through the difficult eight weeks. When my family drank their soup, I'd pour the Modulen into a bowl and drink it with a spoon! Another favourite of mine was making *Modulen ice lollies*! [5]

After the six spoons of heavily-loaded Modulen powder were added to the water, it turned into a rather unappetising gloop before dissolving to form the *liquid* [6]. I therefore advise anyone to find someone else to prepare the drink for them! I was allowed to add a tiny bit of chocolate powder; but this just turned the drink a murky brown colour and hardly altered the taste. If allowed, I'd recommend the chocolate powder anyway to try to trick the brain into thinking that it's a chocolate milkshake! Memories of the smell and taste of the liquid still make me feel sick!

The most difficult part of the diet was that I was a 10-year-old kid, who at the time, just wanted to fit in with everybody else. It was not easy being the only one with a different lifestyle. I had to tell my friends about the diet, because drinking two big cups of brown liquid instead of eating the school lunch looked rather strange. Looking back, I'm not surprised that people had such little understanding of this kind of diet aged 10. I also feel it gave me a lot of strength and courage doing something that was so difficult. As I grew up, I learnt that being different wasn't always a bad thing, especially with the amazing strengths that I developed during this time, which I still recognise seven years later.

4. Alison (dietitian) says:
Brilliant advice to spread the drinks through the day to prevent hunger in order to minimise temptation.

5. Alison (dietitian) says:
Genius!!! These are all great tips which I share with patients

6. Alison (dietitian) says:
Shakers are now available which may help to prevent this happening.

During this time, I was very thankful for my very supportive parents and sister. They all decided to show their support by giving up a food that they love for the duration of the eight weeks. Despite all three of them breaking this promise within a few days, I still knew that they were there to support me *emotionally*! [7]

> **7. Alison (dietitian) says:**
> This demonstrates the importance of having support from those around you including the hospital staff.

Once the eight weeks were finally up, I still couldn't eat my favourite foods, as they had to be reintroduced very slowly. This was because my insides had been given time to calm down, and therefore would have found it difficult to be attacked with salty/acidic/spicy etc. foods all of a sudden. This meant spending about a week eating nothing but the most boring, blandest and dullest foods – plain rice, peeled potatoes, white bread. The first bite of food after eight weeks of nothing but a nasty drink is easy to appreciate, but the novelty soon wore off and it all became very plain. It took a while, but eventually I was back to a normal (sort of!) child who could stuff my face with anything and everything!

I had two more attacks at the ages of 13 and 16, and I am now 17 years old. A year ago, I had the damaged part of my ileum removed through surgery because it had become narrowed, and am now thankfully in remission. I can say from experience that no matter how bad it feels, tastes, or even smells... It does get better!"

Carrie

Carrie is 30 and works as a project manager for a technology company. She was diagnosed with Crohn's disease when she was six years old and would currently describe the severity as 'mild'. Here she talks about her experience of Fortisip and Modulen.

"One of the main treatments I was prescribed during my first admission to hospital was a liquid diet. This diet was prescribed to give my gut a rest and let it heal while the Humira and prednisolone did their job.

In terms of the diet, it mainly consisted of some drinks called Fortisip Compact. These little drinks are only 125ml, and are packed with 300 calories. In order to get

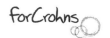

the calories I needed for the day, I was told to drink five of these, in the hope that it would provide me with enough calories to gain some weight.

These drinks went down pretty well at first. The hospital had mostly one flavour, strawberry, but sometimes I would get lucky and get a vanilla one as well. In addition to the Fortisips, I was drinking lots of water and having some clear broths and other liquids, which helped me keep my sanity to a *degree* [8].

After my return visit to the hospital recently, and after feeling quite ill this past Sunday night, the dietitian suggested switching the main calorie component of my liquid diet. So yesterday I started on what is called the Modulen diet. This drink is a bit different, in that it comes in a powder that you have to measure out and mix with water. Not unlike the Fortisip, it comes in a few different flavours. So far I've only tried three: neutral, chocolate, strawberry.

While the drinks themselves aren't necessarily any more palatable, they are much easier to drink, and I think after almost two weeks of Strawberry Modulen, I'm happy to have a change of flavours. I think the drinks also generally settle better in my stomach. After having one, I don't feel like I'm going to explode, and they don't seem to cause much, if any, distress on my digestive system.

The other thing that is neat about the Modulen is that there is more flexibility in how you take it than there was for the pre-prepared Fortisip. I can mix it and drink it normally, or I can freeze it to make ice lollies, or if I fancy a hot beverage, I can warm it up (which I think might be nice with the chocolate and coffee flavours).

The only downside to the Modulen diet, is that to get the most out of it, one is really only supposed to drink the Modulen drinks and water, nothing else. I'm not completely convinced I have the will to do this one, especially for several weeks, but if it adequately relieves my symptoms, I may *stick with it*." [9]

> **8. Alison (dietitian) says:**
> A variety of flavours is good to help what we call "taste fatigue" and so we are always asking the manufacturers of these liquid diets about new flavours in the pipeline.

> **9. Alison (dietitian) says:**
> I am always in awe of patients who follow a liquid diet as it takes an immense amount of effort not to eat or drink anything else. In my experience what spurs people on is that they experience an improvement in symptoms quite quickly. A reduction in pain and having more energy are good motivating factors.

Kelly

Kelly is 28 and married with her first child on the way. She works as a neonatal nurse and was diagnosed with Crohn's nine years ago. Although she would have described her Crohn's as 'severe' a while ago, she is now happily in remission. Kelly talks here about Modulen, the LOFFLEX diet and tips on using a nasogastric tube.

"My first brush with steroids was a good one, I started to feel much better quite quickly. The only trouble came when trying to wean off of them. That's when trying an Elemental diet was suggested. I was 20 by this point, but my dietitian suggested using Modulen (which is normally a paediatric formula). Modulen was actually quite easy to tolerate, although not eating "food" for six weeks was hard. I found keeping a meal routine helpful, making sure I sat at the table with my family and friends at *meal times* [10]. Eating out was actually OK too. It took a little explanation as to why I wasn't eating, but the waiting staff were always understanding and were happy for me to use my own "drinks". It's amazing how you can feel so "left out" when it comes to food and meal times, so trying to keep some normality helps.

> **10. Alison (dietitian) says:**
> This is a really good idea as eating and drinking is such a sociable event and you can feel excluded if you are not eating. However some people find that the smell of food and watching other people eat is difficult and so you need to figure out what works best for you.

The one thing I wasn't expecting was how green my stool would be, it came as a bit of a shock. However my dietitian reassured me that it was completely normal! Phew!

I had an enormous craving for food by the time I finished the six weeks of Modulen, so having to go through a slow exclusion diet to wean back onto food was, well, painful! But it actually went quite quickly, focusing on a food diary and looking out for symptoms took my mind off the timing.

It took a number of months after this to get my symptoms under control, and eventually I weaned off the Prednisolone. My consultant toyed around with different combinations of drugs, firstly trying Budesonide and Sulfasalazine, which had little effect on me. We quickly moved onto azathioprine which helped for a while, but then my liver took a dislike to it, which neatly moved me on to Mercaptopurine.

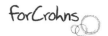

After a period of trying different drugs, followed by some time spent drug-free, I woke up one morning with abdominal pain on my left side, only this time it felt different. The pain took my breath away and worried us both enough to take a trip to A&E. I was admitted into hospital for just under a week with a perforation, but luckily, after lots of tests, it was found that I was having another flare-up. Unfortunately, the inflammation in my small bowel was causing a narrowing, or stricture, which is why it had been so painful. Prednisolone was not helping, so a relatively new drug called infliximab was suggested before I was considered for surgery.

I was placed on another Elemental diet for adults, called E028, and started on the LOFFLEX (Low Fibre, Fat Limited Exclusion) diet. The E028 was much harder to tolerate then the Modulen. In my opinion, it tastes like sick, and I tried having it via *a nasogastric tube (NGT)* [11].

Method for easy *NGT insertion*:

- Hold a cup full of water with a straw, and put the straw in your mouth

- Every time the doctor/nurse pushes the tube over the back of your nose and down your throat, swallow a gulp of water

- *Ask the doctor/nurse to time their pushes with each gulp and swallow* [12]

- If you have to be NBM (nil by mouth), they can then aspirate all the water back out again

> **11. Phil (Gastro) says:**
> NG tubes can be very useful but it is always better to take nutrition by mouth if that's possible.

> **12. Alison (dietitian) says:**
> Great advice as this can be a bit uncomfortable. It sometimes helps to blow your nose beforehand to make sure there is nothing obstructing the passage of the tube

It'll make your eyzes water, but it's a relatively easy way of passing one. Once you've had a few, it might even feel easier to get the nurse/doctor to hold the cup while you pass your own. It makes the timing between pushes and gulps much easier as you're in control. I also used this method to start off an NJT (nasojejunal tube) which I need for an MRI contrast study.

The LOFFLEX diet was much more in depth than any exclusion diet I've tried, and took a few months to complete, but it was well worth it. It helped me understand my food triggers and symptoms associated with this. Although *not all of my symptoms were food-related*, [13] it helped me gain some control and understanding into my condition (as everyone's Crohn's is so different) which will always stay with me."

Travis

Travis is 34 years old, American and a writer. He has had Crohn's disease for nine years and describes it as 'moderate' in severity. Here, Travis discusses his experience of trying to predict which foods might affect his Crohn's.

13. Alison (dietitian) says: This is really important as it is good to be aware that not all symptoms are related to food although at the time it can certainly feel like it. When you have strictures it may not be the food you have just eaten that is causing the symptoms but what you ate yesterday or the day before. This is why keeping a diary during reintroduction can be invaluable.

""You should try this."

"I would, except that would put me in the emergency room. Thanks for trying to assassinate me, Mum. Again."

This is a part of nearly every conversation I have had with my mother since I was diagnosed with Crohn's disease in 2005. Try as I might, I just can't get through to her what my dietary restrictions are. She can't wrap her head around why I can't handle a salad safely, but I can indulge my sporadic craving for White Castle just fine (the pickled onion flavour, if you please). Sometimes, her confusion comes across more like suspicion, as though she's trying to catch me in an elaborate but entirely senseless lie. "Well, how come you can have X?" she'll ask, with that look on her face that says she finds something askance with what I've just told her. If I was still a child, I might be sent to my room just on the basis that my story didn't add up.

It's the convergence of two of our most frustrating issues as Crohnies: diet and being poorly understood by others.

When I grew up as a boy in the 80s, it seemed everyone was healthy. I can still remember the first time I heard about a food allergy. It was sometime in the mid-90s, by which time I was in high school. It sounded like a complete exaggeration to me, or if it was legitimate, so very rare that it was like finding out there was someone out there with pointed ears. It just couldn't be something that affected more than a handful of people, surely.

Today, of course, food allergies are very much a recognised part of the daily lives of many children. It's standard to inquire about them during the admissions process to day care centres, schools or any institution where children will come into contact with food. The assumption has changed. No longer do we take

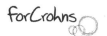

for granted that children are free from those issues. Now we expect that some children face them and must be accommodated.

What sets us Crohnies apart is that our issues are more ambiguous and less consistent. For instance, if you're told that Little Susie has a peanut allergy, then you keep Little Susie away from peanuts. Simple. You can identify the danger and isolate the danger from the potential victim. You also know what the danger is; Little Susie will stop breathing.

For a Crohnie, however, there's no one specific food or ingredient to avoid. Other Crohnies may handle the same foods just fine, on top of that, which can make it especially confusing if someone happens to know two of us. We can make each other seem like liars. "How come Courtney can eat nachos and you can't?" Well, Courtney is a lot luckier than I am, that's why!

I've always shied away from *spicy foods* [14]. Never did I have a taste for things like popcorn or potato chips, either. I hate tomatoes, too. It turns out that all the foods I've naturally avoided are all triggers for me, and/or they pose a very real threat to me in the form of scar tissue and blockages. I think there's something to that, and that's one reason I'm very quick to defend a child who refuses to eat a specific thing. That child may not even understand his or her aversion, but it may come out later that there was a strong physiological reason for it.

14. Phil (Surgeon) says: This is sensible since spicy foods may well lead to looser stools but individuals react differently to different foods and some Crohn's suffers may be able to tolerate spice with no ill effects.

Still, there have been casualties. When it's really hot outside, I sorely miss having a nice, cold salad with some ranch dressing. I miss beer at ball games. (For that matter, I miss ball games!) In the winter, I miss chilli. Every now and again, someone – frequently my mother – will try to goad me into taking the risk and having one of those things. It gives me a great sympathy for recovering alcoholics constantly being tempted by their family and friends. "Oh, one won't kill you. Go on!"

That's the difference between them and us. Their only frame of reference is the periodic tummy ache they've had. At best, they've had food poisoning (yes, I realise I just made it sound like having food poisoning has an upside). For them, though, these are infrequent and very transient aberrations. They pass and then their bodies return to their status quo. They are incapable of understanding that we have to make very specific choices throughout every part of our days.

I have heard of various diets that allegedly help with Crohn's. There are the foods with probiotics, of course. I tried some of the yogurt. I cramped worse than I ever had before and I will not be experimenting with that again. I'm told sauerkraut is rich in probiotics, but its leafy basis scares me. I love 'kraut, though, so occasionally, if I've had a decent stretch of good days and I'm feeling ambitious, I'll risk a little of it. So far, so good, but I live in fear of it just the same. A Crohnie friend of mine has had good luck with the Specific Carbohydrate Diet. Her good news has tempted me to look into it, but as of this writing, I'm still too afraid to venture outside my dietary comfort zone to try it.

That, I think, is the single most important thing about life as a Crohnie: The fear. Every bite we take and every step we take away from a bathroom could be disastrous. I'm afraid to go to restaurants I've never been to before. Even a seemingly obvious dish could be prepared in an unexpected way. It's even likelier that something will be surprisingly unfriendly at someone's home. How am I to know that your grandmother's recipe calls for you to insert walnuts into your mashed potatoes? You've been doing it so long you didn't think to tell me, and it never occurred to me to ask, and now I have to politely decline the dish entirely because your grandmother had the crazy idea to put walnuts in the mashed potatoes.

> **15. Alison (dietitian) says:**
> A lack of understanding can be a very frustrating aspect of having Crohn's disease. Many patients have told me that people think they are fussy eaters or even might have an eating disorder which is easy to say if you haven't got a bowel condition which affects your everyday life.

The best way for me to stay in control of my disease is to have control over which foods to avoid. That's the best I can do. I just wish my mother would quit trying to kill me and *let me continue avoiding them*." [15]

Sally

Sally is 28, has had Crohn's disease for five years and doesn't find that her diet plays too much of an important role in her management of the disease.

"Over the years I have read many books, articles and stories all written by people telling me what I can and can't eat. The truth is, there are only a few real hard and fast rules. As the disease itself is different in each and every person, so are the foods people can eat.

I find as a general rule that high-fibre foods are going to make you go to the loo more. This is a fact. [16] But I have experimented with lots of food that others say

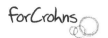

to avoid and been completely fine with it (I have half of my large bowel missing and am on lots of medication, so I don't have the disease mildly!)

16. Phil (Gastro):
This may be true for Sally and some Crohn's patients but not for everyone so find out what 'works for you'.

I really think it's important to test foods yourself. I was so upset that everything I read said 'avoid spicy food' and I am a chilli addict. I still eat chillis now. It might make me go to the loo one more time a day (I don't know exactly, I haven't counted!) but it's worth it. It's not having any detrimental impact on my health. A lot of people also say that they avoid alcohol as it makes them worse; again, I haven't personally found the odd-glass of wine to be a problem, maybe I'm lucky?

I try to have a healthy balanced diet like anyone should. I avoid lentils and chickpeas, because they make me go to the loo more, as does coconut. But in the grand scheme of things, there really isn't that much I need to avoid. Porridge and quinoa are two things that I have found actually work amazingly well for me, against all the advice I had read. They are high-fibre but tend to help 'bulk things out', without being too crude! I eat porridge for breakfast every morning and it really helps, and often have quinoa as an alternative to rice or cous-cous.

I have got to know my own body and figured out what works best for me when it comes to food and drink. I don't want Crohn's to spoil my wonderful relationship with food and I won't let it! I will continue to eat a sensible varied diet, avoiding foods that I know don't work well for me but I will always give them a try before I decide I can't eat them."

Summary

As you've seen, the role of diet in controlling Crohn's can be very powerful, and many people prefer the idea of using diet as a treatment, compared with using drugs. This is particularly true in children, but adults too can benefit from dietary treatments. The difficulty is that they are not too palatable in most cases, so you can see the lengths people go to to improve the taste and tolerability of the diets – it's often quite ingenious! The authors above would argue that the hardships of the diet are worthwhile if a good result is achieved. Normal day-to-day diet can also have an impact, and again we've seen that foods worsening one person's symptoms may be fine for someone else. Each individual will learn their own dietary requirements, and although these stories give

great examples of how diet can help, the specifics will be different for each person.

Tips and suggestions

The tips below come from Alison the dietitian and the stories above.

- **Access to a dietician**
  It is really important that patients have access to advice from a dietitian who has a good knowledge of Crohn's disease and its consequences.

- **Everyone with Crohn's disease is different.**
  You may know someone with Crohn's disease who has been advised by a dietitian to follow a particular diet, but this advice may not be suitable for you.

- **All patients should have their body mass index calculated**
  This should be done at diagnosis to act as a baseline in order to monitor changes in your weight.

- **Get support from your network**
  It is important that friends, family and the whole team looking after the person following the diet are supportive and readily available to give support and advice when difficult circumstances arise.

- **You should never feel silly asking questions**
  All questions are really important and usually have an explanation that can put you at ease.

- **Explore creative ways to consume Modulen**
  Drinking Modulen throughout the day and through straws can make it easier to drink slower and keep you fuller for longer.

  Make Modulen ice lollies or pour it in a bowl and eat it with a spoon like a soup.

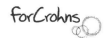

- **Modulen can make your poo green**
  This is normal!

- **Persevere**
  The first two weeks of the diet can be the hardest. Once you settle into a routine, it gets easier.

  Keep a strong positive mental attitude. Try to think of fun ways to get through the difficult times.

Coping with Crohn's disease at work

Having Crohn's can affect your working life in lots of ways. In our experience, it is important to spend time explaining to your employer what effect Crohn's might have on both a day-to-day and a long-term basis. In this chapter, you'll find a number of stories from people about their experiences and tips as to how they handled Crohn's in the workplace.

Crohn's disease from the patients

Kelsea

Kelsea is 22 years old and a student midwife. She was diagnosed aged 20, and has undergone several operations for various aspects of her Crohn's disease. Here she talks about her working life in her previous and current jobs.

"When I was diagnosed with Crohn's disease, I was a full-time student in the final year of a computing degree as well as working as a gym instructor in a local leisure centre. Both the university and my job were already used to me being in considerable amounts of pain; I missed a lot of university and work during

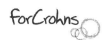

this time, and felt embarrassed to say why. Once I received my diagnosis, I told my university and my job straight away. Both appeared to be very understanding, and work made a plan for me in regards to the job and my health. This allowed me to state any needs I felt I had while there. For example, I was allowed to go and lay down if my backache or stomach pains became too much (within reason, of course). My university gave me extensions on my dissertation and coursework. After my *hemicolectomy* [1], I was off work for eight weeks, as I had an unexpected operation for a perianal abscess during my recovery. When I went back, I had a return-to-work interview, and again this included stating any needs I had in the workplace. I was moved from my gym instructor position to light duties on reception until I felt ready to return to gym instructing. I was allowed to wear my gym instructor uniform on reception (reception uniform was a suit, which was uncomfortable on my stomach) and was put on shorter shifts. Very soon after returning to work, I had another operation *for a fistula* [2].

By this stage, I was very concerned that I would lose my job due to being off so much. However, my work were very understanding. I missed my final exams for my degree, but was offered a degree without honours, as they appreciated the situation I was in. I don't think this was pure luck, as I spoke very openly about Crohn's disease once I was diagnosed, and told my employers and my university what I needed. One of the main issues regarding work life is ignorance; if your employers do not know about the disease, they do not know how to treat you and may just relate it to another condition such as *IBS, and assume you are overreacting* [3].

Out of choice, I am no longer working at that job, as I decided to train as a midwife. *My current university* [4] are also very understanding of my condition, as well as the hospital I work in. Again, I feel this is due to talking about the condition,

1. Phil (Surgeon) says:
Surgery to remove part of the bowel, discussed in more detail in the Surgery chapter.

2. Phil (surgeon) says:
Abscesses and fistula are common in Crohn's and are discussed in detail in the Surgery chapter.

3. Phil (Gastro) and Lucy (IBD) nurse:
Remember, if you need any support in your work place, your IBD Nurse and Gastroenterologist may be able to help with this.

4. Lucy (IBD Nurse):
The key at university is to tell people. You can inform people in the university disability office so you get a room with a toilet on campus, and you may even get access to funds of money to help with your special diet or a parking space nearer campus.

raising awareness, making people realise it isn't just the odd-stomach ache. Crohn's won't beat me and I power through at work as much as I can, which is important! My main piece of advice to others is to remember you have a right to work just like everyone else. Don't use Crohn's as an excuse; however don't let people push you over your limit. Ensure your employers are aware and explain what you need from them so they can get the most out of you."

Gareth

Gareth is 40 years old, married and lives in Birmingham. He has had Crohn's for about 30 years. Here he talks about the serious impact Crohn's has had on his life, and the way he's been able to conquer it - turning his condition into a positive.

"I'll start at the beginning. I had a grumbling appendix. I was 10 or 11. It caused me pain and grief, so they removed it, and for a while it seemed that it grumbled no more – it had been removed after all.

Then when I was 12, despite it no longer being inside me, my appendix was apparently grumbling again! I lost weight; everyone said it was my puppy fat disappearing, but it was dropping off at a relentless pace, and soon I weighed approximately six stone. I looked like a skeleton. AIDS had just begun to appear on TV government warning adverts, and the kids at school decided I had AIDS or cancer, and gave me a hard time.

By the end of the summer, I had been diagnosed with Crohn's disease and put on an extremely high dose of steroids. 80mg. My doctor hadn't had a patient with Crohn's disease before, so I was pretty much his guinea pig. I was the monster to his Frankenstein. I began to get my chubby moon face, my emotions were a rollercoaster and let's not forget the steroidal acne, something you really don't need as you hit your teens.

To be honest, when the specialist said it was Crohn's disease, I always remember that I was pleased, happy as Larry. I'd been so scared of being told I would die, I had Cancer or Aids, that when he mentioned a disease I had never heard of – it sounded a bit funny. If anything I was relieved.

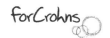

Knowledge is power, so I read up on Crohn's disease. The internet wasn't a big thing at that point (yes, I'm older than I'd like to think, but I don't remember Morse code or gas lamps, so I've got plenty of years ahead of me yet) so you had to do your research. I found National Association of Crohn's and Colitis (now CCUK), and their informative leaflets and books helped further my understanding of my condition.

Steroids were not my best friend, and the dose was ultimately too high. I remember telling people about the horrendous headaches I was getting, and that it felt like my brain was swelling in my head. Everyone thought I was being a drama queen and exaggerating how it felt. We went to my specialist and told him, and his answer to my headaches? "Your brain is swelling in your head!"

Needless to say, my dose of steroids has dropped significantly and we were able to treat my Crohn's reasonably effectively with meds till I was 17. I ended up having emergency surgery and to cut (no pun intended) a very long story short, over the next 13 years, I had more and more bits of Crohn's diseased intestine removed. Most of this happened at my excellent Hospital to whom I am eternally grateful for saving my life on more than one occasion.

> **5. Phil (Surgeon) says:**
> As Gareth says, a jejunostomy is like an ileostomy but from higher up in the small bowel meaning there is less gut between his mouth and his stoma bag in which nutrients and water can be absorbed. People with these high stomas tend to have a high volume output from their stoma and may need nutrition to be given into the vein. This is a very unusual type of stoma and is usually formed when the surgeon has absolutely no other choice because of the problems it causes. Very few people will have this type of stoma but if you're worried then mention it to your surgeon who will almost certainly reassure you that this is not what s/he has planned.

During this time, I managed to go to Southampton Institute, and with support from understanding lecturers, I managed to get a 2:1 for my degree in Film Studies.

After graduating in 1999, I found myself back in hospital as now I had a *Jejunostomy (high output bag from the small intestine* [5]. I mention a Jejunostomy because when I got it, the literature that supported Ostomists (People with Ileostomies, Colostomies and Urostomies) didn't even mention them. Check me out, there I was feeling lonely and isolated, discovering that even the reading materials didn't exist to *support me.*

Eventually I had surgery that I had to ask for, and was relieved when I awoke to discover the bag was gone – although now I had a tube in my chest. This was Total Parenteral Nutrition, because with only 65cm of small intestine left, I was called an Intestinal failure – my new condition was called *Short Gut Syndrome* [6]. Now I had both a disease and a syndrome, I was really gaining nectar points in the world of ill health.

I spent Millennium New Year's Eve in hospital. The Millennium Bug never hit, I became an Uncle (The loudest I've ever screamed in a Hospital and it wasn't from pain) and got my flat done up secretly by my friends so I could come home to a cool pad. On my return to my flat, it's fair to say a depression hit me like no other had before. Dealing with a long-term health condition, especially in your formative years, will inevitably bring about the blues at some or several points. I had battled it during various moments, but stuck in this flat on my own, vomiting every day, hooked up to the nutritional feed through the line in my chest 23.5 hours a day and wetting the bed as a result, I got very *seriously depressed* [7].

I was cold, lonely, unable to drink more than half a glass of fluid a day and couldn't eat without being sick. Long story short, I attempted suicide and was wholly determined to see it through. Through a wonderful quirk related to my health, I was unsuccessful but didn't "fess-up" to anyone until gripped again by intense depression a couple of weeks later.

I'm a lucky man who has the support of good family and friends, and together with some help from them, a psychologist and psychotherapist, I came through the other side.

6. Phil (Surgeon) says:
Short Gut Syndrome is where someone has insufficient bowel to absorb nutrition from food taken by mouth and needs to have it into a vein. The exact length of bowel required to absorb nutrition varies form one individual to another. One key principle of Crohn's surgery is to preserve bowel as much as possible to avoid this problem and it rarely arises. Your surgeon will talk to you about this if it is a risk for you but if you are concerned then mention it so they can allay your fears.

7. Phil (Gastro) and Lucy (IBD Nurse):
Depression is very common in Crohn's disease and not a sign of weakness at all. Please do not suffer in silence and tell your doctor and/or IBD nurse. This is covered in more detail in the Psychological chapter.

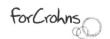

I tried a mixture of jobs until the perfect job presented itself. I'd worked two full-time jobs at 17 and 18 after having to leave school for surgery, but within six months of starting each one, I went through a bad patch with my Crohn's *and lost the jobs due to ill health and being hospitalised* [8]. I found short-term jobs were better for me as there was less of a chance of me getting bogged down and getting ill. I did market research, youth work,

> **8. Phil (Gastro) and Lucy (IBD Nurse):**
> It is sad to hear that Gareth lost jobs due to his illness. We can support people if unwell at work and refer to Occupational Health or you can self-refer.

legal clerking, cartooning, all kinds of jobs that meant I could exist on a freelance basis. When I wasn't well enough to work, I was on income support. There's no shame in claiming benefits. For me, this meant that I could exist without needing to be at home with mum and dad. I fiercely needed my independence so I moved out at 20 and never went back.

Eventually, I started doing stand-up comedy – travelling around the UK by car for the chance to try ten minutes of material in front of a crowd. As time went on, I began to get paid work and in 2005 I did my first solo show, ironically called, "GUTLESS". It was essentially my biopic and the suicide story therein. I took it to the Melbourne international Comedy Festival and got my first lovely review: *"He's cheaper than Prozac and by the end of the show, you feel you've made a friend." Helen Razer: The Age, Melbourne.* I realised there was no reason I couldn't travel all the way to Australia. Now that I had Short Gut Syndrome and Crohn's, it just meant a bit more planning and organising. With my nutritional backpack freaking people out on the plane (mistakenly thinking I was a suicide bomber) and a few questions from customs about all my medical supplies, I was out and about half way around the world. I never thought it would happen.

I then took Gutless to the Edinburgh fringe and got a four-star review in the Metro and more nice quotes. Steadily over the next few years, I built my career, did more solo shows and began to work in ensemble stand-up casts – like Abnormally Funny People (disabled acts) and Cracking Up (acts who've got experience of mental health problems). It takes some resilience to do comedy, but so does having Crohn's and I now feel incredibly lucky to have been able to turn my negative health experiences into funny stories that I can now laugh about (and get paid to tell others).

Now in 2014, I sit in my apartment in Birmingham with my wife Kiruna, and we're working on our careers (I'm still a stand-up, she's an actress) but also on our new company, A Little Commitment, which produces comedy, theatre and workshops..

I've had 14 beautiful years I never expected to have. I got married, built a career and now I'm building a business too, and it's fair to say that without my Crohn's and the ill health – none of those things may have happened.

Looking after yourself emotionally and physically is important too. If you are depressed, find an outlet or people to talk with or to and then take control for yourself.

If physically you need some work, start slowly and build up. Ultimately take charge of your life over the doctors, the friends, the parents and everyone's opinions and find the way to own your health and take control.

What else can I tell you, reader? I can tell you that doctors are not gods, so never be afraid to question, challenge or even doubt their opinion… it's your body they are all talking about, and you're the one who understands how it feels. Also, never give up… I did and it almost cost me my life. Remember, there is a lot of support out there and a lot of people who understand and can help you and finally I'd tell you …Anything is possible with a little commitment. I wish you all the luck and love in the world."

Louise

Louise is 24 years old and works as a shop assistant. She describes her Crohn's as quite severe and was diagnosed two years ago. Here she talks about some of the issues that have affected her since her return to work, following periods of absence due to her Crohn's.

"I am constantly at odds about my job and how it affects my Crohn's, and vice versa.

My primary concern: Not getting sick again.

When I first went back to work, I was about nine weeks out of hospital and finally cleared, but I worried a lot about contact with others. I knew I had a reduced and *compromised immune system*, the last thing I could afford was to go back to work for a couple weeks and be off for another five-month stint. So I was careful. Eventually, I got tired of living in a sort of bubble and becoming paranoid.

In addition to catching something at work, I was also aware of working too much. I work shifts and they can be terrible on my joints – standing up for hours

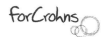

on end, running about, heavy lifting – it would all put pressure on my body. In addition, I was always tired from my *anaemia* [9] and insomnia and would be put down for several consecutive days' work – six days in a row at most. This has happened a couple of times recently, usually including the entire weekend and at least one eight-hour shift. I cannot do that; even now I struggle to make it to the fourth day.

> **9. Phil (Surgeon) says:**
> Anaemia is a low blood count associated with several chronic diseases which reduces the amount of oxygen your blood can carry around making you tire more quickly.

I used to get seriously snippy comments made about my pain and my need to finish work early. I have a very physically demanding job. If I can't do it, the slack falls to someone else. When I was healthy, I could do everything and wouldn't bat an eyelid. Now, I need regular days off and short shifts. Admittedly, I push myself further than I should because I want to prove something; maybe that I'm still the same and I can do the hard stuff that I used to do, that I have not changed, that I am not sick. It's rather stupid, because the fear I felt when I came back – it's still there. It doesn't go away. I have to look after myself, not anyone else. My health comes first, my job second.

I do love my job, I do it really well and hardly ever take a sick day. When it gets too much and my Crohn's acts up through stress and anxiety – even if I don't really feel it to start with – I know I have to step back and stay at home.

My advice? Please listen to your doctor about returning to work. You might feel better and you might be going stir crazy at home, but you are at home for a reason: TO GET BETTER. This means not getting sick again through doing too much or doing something stupid. Being careful is possible at home. At work, people don't really care about your situation; they act like they do, but because Crohn's isn't very well discussed – either through embarrassment or through denial – employers are unaware of how draining it can be, about how your entire life has changed and will continue to change without a moment's notice. But their primary concern is not your health; it is their business, their jobs, their livelihood. Your primary concern? YOUR HEALTH AND YOUR WELLBEING. Take a day off sick. It doesn't hurt anyone. People will cope without you; they did it while you were in hospital and on sick leave.

Next issue: colleagues and your Crohn's disease.

I was so eager to get back to work, I hadn't really thought about how people would react to my new medical condition. In between my third and final admission last year, I went into work for a couple of hours – and everyone came up to me, asked me how I was, commented on how thin I was, how much they missed me, when I would be back, how much I must have gone through. It was nice to have some attention and affection for a while. This all changed once I came back to work.

I thought I would be welcomed back into the work place; and indeed I was, but it was short-lived. I grew quite angry and frustrated at what had been said about me while away: "Oh, she's been in hospital for quite a while, but she's fine now" – FINE?! Really?! Or, even better: "Of course, I know what you're going through, I know someone who has Crohn's". And the kicker? "It's a lot like IBS, isn't it?" I could have screamed when it came to educating people about Crohn's and IBD. I constantly put on a smile and a happy, albeit slightly sarcastic, attitude just to get through the days at work. It is exhausting going back to work: I felt as if I was being re-trained into a job that I had done previously to great ability without fuss. I was treated like a child at times, and then expected to go above and beyond when I was in agony.

One unbelievable moment was being 'disciplined' for taking two days off – weeks apart – when I was physically unable to leave the bathroom at home; this was unacceptable when we all 'need to work as a team'. Apparently, my Crohn's was nothing but a small blip, an inconvenience to the running of the business.

I learnt the hard way on who to talk to about my Crohn's. I have a handful of people who I trust with information about my Crohn's and subsequent treatments and problems. I keep it brief with others who I have learnt not to trust. It bothers me that in a place where I spend most of my time during the week, I can't always be truthful. It is a difficult and very individual situation to explain and talk about.

I know it's all very well for me to sit here, six months back into work, but it's easy to forget that Crohn's changes your life. For me, being in that hospital bed and being at home for all those weeks feels like a lifetime ago. It wasn't even a year ago. It hasn't been that long and there are symptoms that you just can't control or predict. Even I – someone who is kept healthy with a biological medication – need time to just not work. I am no longer like my colleagues; I can't be the super woman I used to be. I can't do it all. And some days, I just need reminding: IT'S JUST A JOB."

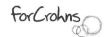
John

John is 55 years old, married and a father. He is a writer but previously worked in marketing. He has suffered from Crohn's for more than three decades and has undergone several operations during that time. He is now in remission and has written a book about his experiences ("The Foul Bowel: 101 Ways to Survive and Thrive with Crohn's disease") from which he has adapted this extract.

"Walking out of the hospital following my diagnosis of Crohn's and news of impending surgery, my mind wandered to what would prove to be the most difficult part of succeeding at being ill: How do you combine an on-going illness with the need to build a career or, at the very least, remain in paid employment? What would this mean back in the workplace? What should I tell my new boss when I returned to the office the next day? "I'm going to be off work for I don't know how long, commencing I don't know when" would not be too welcome and equally not much use to him in planning around my absence.

So prolonged was my absence due to be – 12 to 16 weeks - that the work clearly could not be allowed to pile up for my return, nor could it reasonably be doled out to my colleagues to cover. If it was for three or four weeks, then maybe they would muddle through, but three or four months meant that I had to come to terms with the fact that someone else would be doing my job and it may not be there for me when I returned.

The meeting went well. It was made clear to me that all that mattered was my health and that they would cope. We agreed that the job would have to be done full-time by someone else and that, closer to my return date, we would have to discuss other possible vacancies. I have since met many fellow sufferers who ended up losing their jobs because of the amount of time they were taking off, and many had found it very difficult to get back into the workforce. I was lucky that I was working in a large enough organisation where I was a very small cog in a very large wheel, so my absence would not sink the ship.

If your absences could cripple your employer, I believe it is unreasonable of you to expect them to bear such a burden. Get yourself into as large an employer as possible. Even if you have to compromise your ideal job to be with an employer where your absences can more easily be borne, it is a compromise worth making.

Even so, it was a very big frustration that I was unable to tell my employer when this prolonged absence would commence. I understand that, especially these days, scheduling of surgery is a day-to-day process a s they strive for 100 per cent bed occupancy rates, but if I could change one thing about the health profession, it would be to get them to *realise that you have a life and a career* [10] too, and that you don't have as much flexibility as they seem to imagine.

After the surgery, I focused myself on my other key priority: that of planning the future direction of my career. My thinking began as follows: The hardest thing to come to terms with when dealing with Crohn's would be that it does not go away. Hence, my life was most likely going to be a series of ups and downs where, in the down periods, I would be juggling the options of drug regimes, surgery, putting up with feeling ill, or sometimes all three simultaneously. It would clearly be a mistake to add to this burden by over-stretching myself in the workplace.

> **10. Phil (Surgeon) says:**
> I think this is a fair comment and most units will try to accommodate work schedules and holiday dates and so on where possible, but surgeons mostly operate on the same one or two days a week and their operating lists are often filled months in advance with other patients all wanting the same slots and also with a strong argument to be done asap. Discuss scheduling with your surgeon to see what they can do to help but don't expect miracles.

Having had a few weeks to think about things, and bearing in mind the prognosis on the probable future course of my health, I came to the conclusion that I would be foolish to continue my immediate career path as a brand manager in the marketing department.

Jobs that depended on lots of doing – and brand management was a good example – would just be setting me up for a fall. Stress makes illnesses worse and being a brand manager was close to being one of the most stressful jobs in a company like Cadbury. You initiate things and have to follow them through to execution, usually multiple projects at once – plenty of ball-juggling. Also, the advertising agencies were in London, so that meant every week there would be one or two long days' travelling together with heavy-duty lunches. If, in the future, I was to feel as ill as I had done in the preceding months, then these responsibilities and punishing schedules would just pour fuel on the fire.

When feeling ill, I would feel compelled to struggle into work if my absence would mean things grinding to a halt or going wrong. I did not want to do this, as it would, I was now convinced, ultimately shorten my life. Conversely, if I took the time off when I was under the weather, I would ultimately fail in the job.

The question that was top of my mind was: given that Crohn's disease was for life and had already shown the level of disruption it could bring into the workplace, was there an alternative career path where I would be better able to shield the company from the new limitations I was now probably going to face? In other words, assuming the worst health-wise, how could I prevent my illness from making my employment a problem for the company and consequently for myself? But if not marketing, then what? I had been pondering these questions almost since the day I had left the hospital, but the direction I needed to take was increasingly clear: I needed to be able to work when feeling ill.

I believe that with an illness like Crohn's, one should look for a job that you can comfortably do when you are feeling well and get by in when you are feeling ill. Do not get into jobs where you are fully stretched when you are feeling well as you will surely fail when your health is poor. It is better to over-achieve in a role you are comfortable in rather than fail in a too demanding role.

The best kind of role for me was one that depended primarily on the quality of my thinking rather than the energy of my doing. No matter how bad I was feeling, and whether I was in the office or tucked up in bed, I could still think. This inevitably led me back to the area where I had started my career, which was much more of a thinking role. In the market analysis department, the key areas of added value were gleaning insights into reasons behind past sales performance that could be applied by colleagues in the marketing department to positively influence the future. I felt confident that I could definitely do well in that role whatever the state of my health. Plus, going back into an area I was familiar with would enable me to ease myself back into the workplace once my sick leave had run its course. So I called the personnel department and set up a meeting to discuss options for my return.

The bottom line was that I was prepared to take a step back in my career in the short term to have more control over its direction, no matter what the illness would throw at me. I was only 25 years old; I needed a long-term plan that would enable me to build a career for the next 35 years while avoiding having to choose between health and career.

With Crohn's, you have to plan much further ahead than you did in the past and more so than others do. I have met countless people for whom Crohn's has effectively taken control of their future, simply because they carried on as before they were ill and hoped for the best. Plan for the worst and treat anything better than that as a bonus. Stay in control of your destiny.

25 years later, I believe my thinking was correct."

Summary

Within these stories, you would have found a range of experiences and perspectives about how to manage Crohn's in the workplace. Every individual has different priorities and while for some, a career is low on their priorities, for others this might be very different.
One important element of managing your Crohn's within the workplace is to be aware of your rights as an employee.

Employee rights and Benefits

Further information can be found on the Crohn's and Colitis UK website, upon searching for employment, but here is a concise summary taken from this site:

Nearly all workers have certain legal rights and you may have additional rights in your particular employment contract. You can obtain further information about general employment rights from several sources including the government website: www.direct.gov.uk, ACAS, Citizens Advice and trade union representatives.

Having Crohn's, you may be particularly worried about whether your employer can dismiss you for ill health. The law does give some protection here, but the level of protection will depend on whether you are treated as disabled under the Equality Act 2010.

If your Crohn's is considered a disability, your employer has a legal duty to make 'reasonable adjustments'. Dismissal because of a disability may be unlawful discrimination. You may have grounds for bringing a claim for disability discrimination even if you do not have one year's service. The Equalities Act 2010 defines disability as a physical or mental impairment that has an effect on a person's ability to carry out normal day-to-day activities. This includes 'hidden' impairments or disabilities such as incontinence. The effect must be substantial, adverse and long-term.

If the Equality Act applies to you, you can ask your employer for reasonable adjustments when any aspect of your working arrangements, including the building or place of work or your working hours, puts you at a substantial disadvantage compared to a non-disabled person doing your job. These adjustments are not favours but rights.

Helpful adjustments that would not generally be too expensive could include:

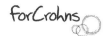

- Allowing time for medical appointments or treatment

- Changes to your working day such as shorter or different hours

- Unlimited toilet breaks

- Moving your work station close to a toilet

- Providing a car parking space close to the entrance into work

- Allocating some of your duties to someone else

- Offering another place of work

Where adjustments are expensive, such as installing separate toilet facilities, a scheme called Access to Work may be able to help.

Ultimately, if it is not possible for you to agree with your employer about whether an adjustment is reasonable, you could issue a claim in the employment tribunal in respect of your employer's failure to make reasonable adjustments and seek an award of damages. However, before you are able to issue a claim, you would need to raise a formal written grievance with your employer. Contact the Equality and Human Rights Commission for further information

Benefits: Fast facts
Another important element to managing a career with Crohn's disease is to understand the impact Crohn's might have on your financial situation. It might therefore be useful to investigate the possibility of claiming benefits to support yourself.

The benefits system is complex and frequently changes. For up-to-date basic information you might like to refer to the government website GOV.UK www.gov.uk/browse/benefits

Crohn's and Colitis UK produce a guide *'An Overview of Welfare Benefits for People with Ulcerative Colitis and Crohn's disease'* and have a helpline for support with benefits advice and applications.

The key benefits to consider are:

Attendance allowance is a benefit payable to people, aged 65 and over, who have a health condition which has lasted at least six months.

Disability Living Allowance (DLA) changed to Personal Independence Payments **(PIP) from 8 April 2013.** PIP is designed to help people aged 16-64 meet the extra costs that come from having a long-term health condition or disability. For the purposes of PIP, a long-term condition means ill-health or disability that is expected to last 12 months or longer. PIP is made up of two parts (components), a Daily Living component and a Mobility component. Each component has two rates; standard and enhanced. PIP isn't affected by income or savings, it's not taxable and people can get it whether they're in or out of work.

Employment and Support Allowance (ESA) is a benefit which is payable to people who are unable to work due to ill health or disability. It replaced Incapacity Benefit (IB) in October 2008.

Tips and suggestions

- **Don't be shy about admitting that you suffer from Crohn's:**
  If you're an office worker and you need to sit at a desk closer to a toilet, ask.

  If you are running late because you couldn't leave the bathroom, then be honest (not in so many words, no one needs explicit details!).

  Having a long-term condition means that you will need more doctors and hospital appointments than most. Again, make sure your employer is aware of why you are going to see the doctor. You might have a dermatologist appointment one week, one with your gastroenterologist the next and then one with an IBD nurse the following week. If your employer is strict, you could provide them with copies of your appointment letters to prove where you are going and why, or ask the doctor you see to produce a letter saying where you were but without

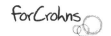

the details of why you were seen, since these are confidential and no one else's business. This takes very little time and is a small request to make. Don't underestimate how long these appointments take either. It is better to say that you are going to be gone for the afternoon than to say you'll be back in an hour. Hospitals generally overbook clinics and run late, so be aware that you might take longer than you anticipated.

- **If you are on drugs such as infliximab or adalimumab, that lower your immune system, make sure that your employer understands this.**
  You may well get more colds than most people in your workplace and you may want your employer to understand why.

- **The key is if you think that your Crohn's symptoms are affecting how well you are able to do your job, tell your employer.**
  Keep them informed and educate them. Remember, the more people who know about Crohn's disease and understand it, the better. Don't be shy, don't be embarrassed, just be ready to educate.

- **Look out for the practical steps you can take to make working easier for you**
  If you're less worried and less inconvenienced by your Crohn's, you'll be more productive and both you and your employer will notice the difference.

Having a relationship when you have Crohn's disease

Crohn's will make relationships difficult at some stage in everyone's life, whether with a partner, friends or relatives – perhaps all of them at some point! It is important to try and tell those closest to you how you are feeling so they can at least try and begin to understand. This chapter examines how Crohn's can have an impact on your relationships, how to try to minimise this and how it might even bring you closer together with some people.

Crohn's might put a strain on your relationship with your partner, both physically and emotionally. It is important to let your partner in and tell them how you are feeling. Remember they are more than likely feeling helpless and struggling to see you in pain, so bear with them if they seem frustrated sometimes. During a flare-up or after surgery, it is unlikely you will want to be intimate with your partner, but make sure that they feel loved in other ways. Problems will arise from you not communicating with your partner, so keep telling them how you're feeling.

It may also have an effect on your friendships. Friends might not understand why you can't come out when you are having a flare-up. Again, this is where you need to communicate or suggest doing something that doesn't involve eating or drinking. Spending time in your own home, where the loo is close, is always an option. Remember good friends want to see you and spend time with you, regardless of what you are doing or where you are.

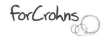

Crohn's does not have to dictate who you are. It might dictate what you have to do from time to time, but make sure you can still see your friends when you want to. Don't shy away.

Crohn's disease from the patients

Sally

Sally is a 28-year-old woman who has had Crohn's disease for five years. She tells her story of informing dates about her Crohn's and meeting her boyfriend.

"After being in a relationship for many years, I found the idea of dating daunting enough, never mind the fact that I also have Crohn's and have a temporary ileostomy.

It was something I considered very carefully for quite some time before joining the dating scene again. Unfortunately there is no rulebook for dating anyway, so I think you just need to follow your gut (excuse the pun).

The first man I told was after about four dates. We were getting to the stage where I felt that I trusted him and I wanted to tell him so he knew more about me, and obviously it's not something you can hide if you want to have a physical relationship with someone! I found it so difficult to get the words out of my mouth that I scared him into thinking I was going to tell him the most hideous thing imaginable – the way I was crying and couldn't look at him. Then when I told the story of my Crohn's, from start to finish, and explained that this ileostomy had saved my life, his exact words, were "is that all? I thought you were going to say something really bad". Things with him went on for a little longer, but didn't progress in the end, though I knew it wasn't down to my illness or my ileostomy – it was down to us not being compatible.

That is one important thing to remember when you are dating with a chronic illness. We can all sometimes be too quick to blame the Crohn's for problems in our lives, but sometimes relationships will fail for many other reasons other than having Crohn's, or having an ileostomy.

I had a similar situation with another man that I was dating. After five dates, I decided it was the right time to tell him my whole sorry story from diagnosis to operations. He was really touched that I felt comfortable enough to tell him all of this and was really understanding. What I find really fascinating is that both men I'd told felt that they needed to tell me something that had happened to them, too. A big, deep dark secret about them or their family. It's interesting how everyone has some kind of secret, it might not be an illness, but unfortunately no one lives a perfect life without any problems and I've started to realise that more and more since dating.

The third man I told is my now boyfriend. We clicked instantly after our first date and I felt I could tell him anything and everything. Obviously I waited a few more dates before telling him, but there weren't as many tears and I managed to look him in the face as I told him everything. Maybe that's because I'd had the practice of saying it all a couple of times before, or maybe it's because I was telling someone I knew I was truly starting to care about. He told me straight away that if things continued in the way they were that he would be there to support me through any reversal operations, or any operations to make it permanent. He made me feel like none of that mattered. It doesn't make you less attractive, in many ways, it can make you more attractive. It shows a strength of character that you have overcome such troubled times. It shows that you can be brave and that you're a fighter. It also means that I don't tend to 'sweat' the small things in life so much. In many ways, having a chronic illness has turned me into a better person and therefore a better potential partner for single men out there.

My only piece of real dating advice would be – don't be ashamed of who you are and the illness that you have. Don't talk about it in a negative way to potential partners. Tell them about the battles that you've had, but explain how you've overcome them. Explain how having Crohn's doesn't define you as a person. It's part of being you, but it's not all-consuming. Don't feel you need to tell someone everything on a first date. You don't. Open up about everything when you feel ready and comfortable. Don't always expect the reaction you want, but anyone worth continuing a relationship with will listen and be caring. It's a good test of someone's compassion in many ways.

Most importantly, enjoy the dating experience. Remember, no one is perfect and you have nothing to be ashamed of."

Travis

Travis is a 34-year-old man who has had Crohn's disease for nine years. He tells his story of the impact of Crohn's on his relationship and finding a new partner.

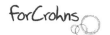

"When I was diagnosed, I had already spent two years with the woman I would marry. She knew what I was like before Crohn's disease derailed my plans and imposed new, unfair limitations on me. She could anchor herself to that memory of who I was. It sustained us for several years until I could no longer tolerate the difference in myself and I slipped into a year-long bout of severe depression that ultimately cost me my marriage. This is probably pretty ominous sounding, so let me just say: don't freak out!

I found myself in a very peculiar place after my marriage disintegrated. I hadn't given any thought to ever having to meet someone else. The last time I met someone was my wife, and that was before Crohn's. How would I explain the disease? Or account for why I'm not at the same kind of place that my peers are, or even my own friends? How could I sell myself, with the baggage of Crohn's disease?

I eventually signed up with some online dating services. I floundered on all of them, I think primarily because I'm not the kind of guy who does well in that kind of environment. It's just not in my nature to message a woman I know nothing about and see if she wants to meet for drinks (the fact that Crohn's is incompatible with drinks is immaterial). I put it on a mental backburner for a while, not really expecting any progress. A local theatre hosted a midnight screening of The Man with the Golden Gun and some of my friends who share my enthusiasm for James Bond films decided we'd go. Lo and behold, my guts cooperated and I was able to attend that night. One friend brought a co-worker with him. She and I hit it off immediately.

I confess that I was intimidated about how to proceed. I didn't want her perception of me to be predicated on my diagnosis. That was one of the things that really bogged me down during my Year of Hell with depression; I had come to feel that I was a condition to be monitored rather than a human being. I needed her to see me as a human being and not a diagnosis. Still, there are practical implications to life with Crohn's. If we set a dinner date, for instance, I would need her to understand why it couldn't be at, say, a Cajun or Indian restaurant. Or why I might spend half the dinner in the bathroom, or not make it at all. The last thing I needed was her to think I had stood her up!

The decision was kind of taken out of my hands anyway because, unbeknownst to me, she had found and begun reading my blog after we met at the movie. She was able to glean from that enough about my experiences with both Crohn's disease and depression that she had a pretty good sense of what my daily life was like before we ever discussed such matters. It was something of a cheat, I suppose, but we still had "The Talk". I had to tell her how afraid I was every time

I went to the bathroom that it might be the first red flag telling me a trip to the emergency room was in order. How I hate driving because the random nature of distracting pain terrifies me. Why I've stopped going to concerts or any event with lots of traffic and crowds between me and a bathroom. I'm not going to go on a white water rafting getaway weekend.

I have rarely felt more vulnerable than I did when she tentatively asked about what living with Crohn's meant for me. I thought of all the conversations I've had over the years, even recently, in which women have scoffed at guys who were interested in them but offered no financial security or seemed too much of a homebody. There are standards every woman ought to have, you see… and I was effectively asking a woman to not hold me to them. I thought about our gender-based double standards as a society and I honestly don't know which is worse. It's much more accepted for a male to have digestive woes than it is for a female. In this, I felt a pang of sadness for my Crohnie sisters who have to face a stigma that, fortunately, I'm able to more or less circumvent.

However, I think there's also still a greater expectation placed on men to be breadwinners – even by women who are entirely self-sufficient. "I don't want to have to take care of him!" is a common refrain among women explaining why they have rejected a potential suitor. Not only am I not a breadwinner, but I have to be careful about even eating that bread, lest I really need someone to take care of me!

Many people are self-conscious about their bodies. We fixate on our perceived flaws; that's universal. As a Crohnie, there's more to fret over than merely not having washboard abs. Our abs may be scarred, sometimes severely, from various surgeries. It's not uncommon for a Crohnie to be uncomfortable being shirtless, even during sex. Plus, there's the fact that under the skin, our guts are trying to sabotage us.

Sex is like performing live on stage; it requires a certain suspension of self-awareness. Crohn's is a heckler armed with sounds and smells and you hope it was too preoccupied to come to tonight's show. Abdominal activity is obviously questionable for us Crohnies. Even just doing sit-ups can be terrifying g, much less performing the kind of gyrations that occur during sex. Each movement can bring us closer to rousing the attention of our heckler, who can ruin the mood entirely.

I've had to stop abruptly to run to the bathroom more than once. Talk about a mood killer! No matter how good one's hygiene, there's something about coming directly out of the bathroom that discourages sexual intimacy for many (probably most) of us. Then there are the medications. Prednisone is funny, because it has

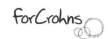
definitely been known to boost my libido. Yet the more I've taken of it, the worse my hips and my back have become. After a few years of living with frequent *Prednisone tapers* [1], sex became a race against my own body. How long could I go before it simply hurt too much to continue? Sometimes, not long at all. I wouldn't care to rank them, but I have often felt even more self-conscious about having to stop because my body hurts than because I had to run to the bathroom. I don't know why that is, except maybe that it's part of that "invisible illness" thing. At least when my bowels erupt, there's evidence of why our *lovemaking has to cease* [2].

> **1. Phil (Surgeon) says:**
> This is where you slowly wean off steroids to avoid problems that can occur if you stop too suddenly after a prolonged course. See the Drugs chapter.

Of course, even just being in the mood can require an act of Congress on a day when Venus is in the right retrograde. Life with Crohn's involves a whole lot of being run down and feeling tentative. It gives one a sense of what it must be like to be an active, though irregular, volcano. Provided I can even muster the energy to want sex, there's the other matter of whether I feel it's reasonably "safe"

> **2. Phil (Gastro) and Lucy (IBD Nurse):**
> A full and active sex life is possible with Crohn's disease, even with a stoma. The most important factor is finding a partner you feel close enough to share your difficulties with – a person who will understand how Crohn's disease affects you on a daily basis.

to try. Of course, even all that is only half of the equation, because should I get a green light from my own body, there's the matter of my partner.

I've always been more disappointed if I'm the holdup. I've been the one who wasn't up to it enough that I feel empathy for my partner if it's her night to not feel it. Conversely, I feel guilty if it's my fault. I won't hesitate to tell you that's a bunch of nonsense and you shouldn't feel guilty for not wanting sex, but since I'm being honest, that's how I feel even knowing it's not fair to me."

Wendy

Wendy is 49, married with one child and works as a writer. She was diagnosed with Crohn's when she was 19, has had many operations and would describe her Crohn's as 'moderate-severe'.

"I'd known my boyfriend for a while before we started going out, so he knew about my Crohn's, and he also knew I wasn't into serious relationships and I didn't 'do' commitment. I'd made all that very clear when he'd finally convinced me to be

his girlfriend. I'd told him quite a lot about my disease and how I'd already had three surgeries and was very likely to need more. I explained what it was and how it worked and how it had affected me, but it was all fairly abstract. All he'd really seen was that I had to go to the toilet a lot, and that I took copious amounts of *Codeine* [3].

So it was probably a bit of a shock when, after an ill-advised Chinese dinner that wasn't supposed to have any MSG in it, my 'casual' boyfriend of just three months had to rush me into hospital and wait five and a half hours for me to come out of emergency surgery for an obstruction. During those fraught hours, he met my mother and sisters for the first time.

And then he came to visit me daily. Really. Every day, as I lay in the hospital. Once the anaesthetic had worn off properly and I'd started to give it some thought, I realised this wasn't entirely fair on him. Don't get me wrong; I liked it, it was great, but I wasn't sure it was what he really wanted to be doing. I wondered if maybe he was just too decent a person to admit that he wanted out. After all, it wouldn't look that great, would it? A guy leaving his girlfriend while she was sick in hospital, recovering from major emergency surgery; I could see why he hadn't done it. But I really didn't want him to feel that he couldn't, shouldn't, or mustn't. So one evening I told him not to come the next day. He looked like I'd punched him in the stomach. If he was going to stay away from me, that would be his decision, he told me. If I wanted rid of him, then I should just say so, as he wasn't in any hurry to go anywhere. I ended up following him down to the lobby, telling him he didn't need this, and I wasn't about to force him into coping with it. I was shouting at him before long; making a big scene in a reception area which swarmed with people, all with their own reasons for being in the lobby of a London teaching hospital; all far too busy to notice somebody else's drama unfolding. Which meant nobody interrupted us, or asked us to keep it down. I yelled at him that I'd coped my whole life on my own; just me and my Crohn's. I didn't need somebody else to look after me; I wasn't looking to share the load. It was my load, and I was more than used to it. We'd had a lovely time together; it had been great while it lasted – Chinese MSG free meal excepted – and we should leave it like that: as a nice, perfect, finished thing that we'd both enjoyed and that was now over. I had plenty of friends and family to help me out, and I wasn't expecting or asking him to watch

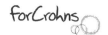

me get sicker and sicker and feel like he had to stay so that he didn't seem like some kind of bastard. He should just go, I told him; there'd be no hard feelings, and he could go back to his life the way it was before he met me.

The door was there, in front of us; all he had to do was go through it, I could go back to my side-room on the ward, and we'd say no more about it. But he wasn't interested in walking away. He didn't want to go back to his old life; he didn't want to leave me on my own. He hadn't walked into this relationship with his eyes closed any more than I had.

A fire alarm went off while we were arguing. Patients in gowns drifted down into the lobby, with hospital staff reassuring them that it wasn't a real situation; that the alarm had gone off by accident. And still we stood there – me in my hospital gown, dragging a drip-stand and *TPN* bag along behind me, and him with the bright sunshine lighting him into silhouette as he refused to leave.

The thing is, I wasn't trying to get rid of him because I didn't give a toss about him. I was trying to protect him, and I'll be honest – I was trying to protect myself, too. I didn't want him to walk away; of course I didn't. I just thought he should. While I was still perfectly able to manage things alone, as I always had. This was when he should leave; before I became dependent on him, and couldn't let him go. Before I got so sick that he would hardly be able to leave my bedside, because that was what surely lay ahead. The way my particular disease worked, historically, this first visit to the hospital; this first experience of emergency surgery; of wondering if I'd be alive the next time he saw me; this first go at all of this was just that – the first go. I wasn't going to get better; I was going to get worse. My doctors all said that; they knew it. I'd had all the surgeries that were supposed to 'cure' me. Or at least put me in remission. And they'd failed. Here I was now, a sufferer who would continue to suffer. There'd be more surgeries; more bits removed; inevitably a bag would appear sooner or later, and finally … well, who knew? But if he was going to stay with me, he needed to consider the worst-case scenario; he needed to think about whether he could handle it. I said he should take some time; that I wouldn't be angry if he decided to call it a day. He said he'd already spent quite enough time thinking about it, and that he wasn't going anywhere. It was up to me whether or not I believed him, but he was happy to spend the foreseeable future proving it. How does a person argue with that? It's a shame that everyone was too busy with their own dramas to notice ours; when we hugged and declared ourselves in love with each other, a round of applause would have been good.

And just so you know, it's now 24 years later; we've been married for 21 of those, have a healthy 19-year-old son, and I've had an ileostomy for the last 20 months. It's all going well so far!"

Louise

Louise is 24 and in a long-term relationship. She has had Crohn's for a year and a half and talks about having an ex with the condition before her own diagnosis, as well as being intimate with Crohn's.

"My connection with Crohn's disease didn't begin with my own diagnosis, but many years previous to that with my first serious boyfriend. I was 18 at the time, when one weekend in February he was rushed into hospital needing an emergency bowel resection. They removed quite a large chunk of his small bowel, resulting in short gut syndrome and a very lengthy and frustrating hospital stay. I am the first to admit that I was scared, and I wasn't even the patient.

I spent some time off from university taking care of him during his six-week recovery period. It was tough – the scar, for one – from diaphragm to the lower belly. *The medication. The pain* [4]. The emotional turmoil of being in a relationship with someone who was sick was tough too. I have spent a lot of time in the years since we broke up 'erasing' this period in my life – I wasn't always so loving and caring about his condition – but in September 2011, I got my karma. I was diagnosed with Crohn's disease myself. I spent six weeks in hospital over four separate visits in the space of three months. I went through the rounds of medications, tests and scans to eventually receive a treatment that worked for me; giving me my 'normal' life back.

It was February this year that I met my now current boyfriend. We've only just started dating, but there is nothing that he doesn't know about my condition. We were great friends – I'd even go as far to say best friends – before we even contemplated a relationship. I made the conscious choice after my time spent in hospital to be open and honest about my condition with people, even new ones in my life. He is a tremendously caring and understanding person. I know that he thinks my condition is scary – who wouldn't? – but he sees my bravery and courage before anything else.

> **4. Phil (Gastro):**
> This is a normal feeling that particularly young people describe. However, many realise that without the scars, and the battles that they have faced, they would not be the people they are. Those who have had to have a stoma may not even be alive or be able to function without it, so accepting it is part of you and learning how to live with it is a useful goal.

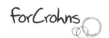

We met through a mutual friend. I wasn't even consciously looking for anyone, so at some point during our first meeting I spoke the words that cause every Crohnie some sort of dilemma: "I have Crohn's disease". I am lucky – he knew about it already. But being a very individualistic condition, he did not know about the Humira, about my own battles I've had to fight and ones I still battle. It was a couple weeks later, after spending quite a few nights together hanging out that he broached the subject again: "So, tell me about these injections you have to take and why they are so damn wonderful". I explained. I talked a lot that night. About my hospital stays, about the medications that I had tried, why Humira was so important and so amazing and why I was now 'healthy'.

Having spent my time in hospital without any friends around me, I was surprised at my level of chatter. About how open I was with him about my condition. I didn't see him as anything but my friend. Someone to vent to when times got rough – this happened a lot in the first month of being friends – and someone I could occupy my time with, to keep me busy and my mind off the disease. He always took – and takes – a keen interest in anything I have to say about my Crohn's. I nicknamed my guts and he was there with me. He embraces and encourages the quirky things about me, the very silly and humorous things I do.

Why did I share it all with him, despite just being friends? I don't really know a solid answer for this one. A big part of me shared with him because, at the time, I was burdening myself with a lot of my own issues; there was no one there to talk to. Another big part of me talked to him because he asked. No one else did at that stage. They are both interlinked. But mostly I shared with him because I knew he was a good man; that I could be myself, my whole Crohnie self with him.

But despite being open with him, and the fact that I have no scars from my Crohn's, I do try and keep some boundaries. I inject myself with Humira every two weeks. I do that alone, always. I do not want to share that with him just yet. I try my best to hide my little Crohnie belly from him – the 'chubby' fat bit of my stomach – and I try not to see him when I am exhausted from work and stressed. But being friends before our relationship meant that I could share with him things I would find difficult if I had just dated him. Such as: my horrible scopes and scans, the blood tests, the side-effects of my long list of failed medication, my emotional 'denial' of Crohn's, my depression, my anger. It was very easy to talk to him about everything and anything that bothered me. And because of that, we have a much closer relationship now. I would not have got into any sort of relationship that meant my Crohn's became an 'issue' – it is not an excuse or something to blame things upon, that is unfair and uncalled for – and I would never get involved with someone who didn't understand or care about me and my health.

I was slightly concerned about how I was ever going to have another relationship again when they diagnosed me with Crohn's. I openly admit I worried more about how I was going to be naked in front of another human being, a boyfriend, a fiancé, a husband, than I did my scary list of medications.

Why? Because part of it is just a natural reflex. I knew that my Crohn's meant and will mean surgery and scars. And that is something I have to deal with when it comes, but the symptoms and side-effects of my Crohn's disease make it more of a challenge to be with someone in a real way. I say "challenge" because "problem" reeks of something negative; and as if you are the issue that doesn't make things 'work' out like they should have or would have done if you were illness-free.

It took me a long time as a teenager and as a young adult to feel comfortable in my skin. And I won't let my Crohn's disease take that away from me. My current boyfriend knows that. Not rushing into anything physical was the first ground rule I established. It was difficult, because when you like someone, you want to be with them in every single way you can think of, and holding off on that was torture, but good for us. Leaving it longer would have made it worse, so there needs to be a happy medium – discussed by both of you – of when you can display your physical desire for one another.

Having sex for the first time since my diagnosis was many things. It had been about six months, and the first thing I felt was relief. It was good to know that my body wasn't as bad as I thought it was, and that someone wanted me as much as I wanted them. It was good to know that some things about me were still very normal. During my depressive months, I felt completely unattractive and completely devoid of any sex drive; to have that come back was great – amazing, in fact. It was also uplifting. All the things I feared before were suddenly very unimportant and stupid, petty even. I won't lie and say there aren't moments when I get a lovely tummy rumble or we have to stop half-way through because I feel awful and need the sanctuary of a bathroom, but on the whole it makes me feel good. I know that inside of me, I used to have a torrent of pain and inflammation, but I feel none of that anymore.

Like jumping into the ocean, only you will know when you are ready to take the plunge. Just don't take every embarrassing thing too seriously and laugh. Just be... happy.

Having Crohn's is a complicated thing. If you are lucky enough to have avoided depression alongside your medication issues, great! But I do have to deal with my depression, along with my Crohn's, work, my family and now a new boyfriend. Having a relationship with Crohn's isn't easy. It's as much work, if not more, when you have an incurable condition. Add in the fact that it can flare up without notice

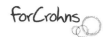

and can result in a lot of hospital time; it is tough. But there IS someone out there who will love you just as you are. Who won't care if you don't always feel up for going out, who will be happy just staying in, who will support you through everything medical-related, who will cheer you up with silly gestures when you feel down. There is someone who will adore you because of your disease. They will see how wonderful and special you are because of everything you've been through. Want to know a little secret? You are so damn worth it."

Summary

Relationships are hard work whether you have Crohn's or not. These stories show that it is possible to have a happy, fulfilling relationship regardless of your disease. In fact, in some cases, it can even bring you closer together. Our authors seem to suggest that honesty is the best policy; open up and let your partner know how you are feeling and what to expect when you're having a bad day and how they can help.

Tips and suggestions

- **Communicate**
  Let people in and tell them how you are feeling; they are not mind readers and often, if they realise what you're feeling, they will be more understanding.

- **Timing**
  Although it is important to communicate with people, you can do this in your own time, you don't need to tell them everything the first time you meet them and can keep some things back if you want to. Don't tell people until you are ready to and choose the setting, atmosphere and context yourself. Leave yourself plenty of time to discuss it, as they may have lots of questions. Remember their reaction may not be the one you're expecting, so be prepared for either a long discussion or a rapid change of subject. Have a longer talk some time in future, when they've had a chance to think about it.

- **Don't be ashamed of who you are and the illness you have.**
  Everyone has bits of their life that aren't perfect. Crohn's is certainly part of what you bring to a relationship but it is only a part – the rest of what makes you 'you' is much more important.

  If you are sat worrying what the other person thinks of you, whether they will like you, whether they think you're attractive and so on, don't forget that they're wondering the exact same things, albeit for a different reason.

Having children when you have Crohn's disease

Crohn's disease often affects women during the period of their life when they are likely to want children. This raises many questions about whether it is safe to get pregnant: whether a Crohn's disease flare-up is likely to occur during pregnancy, whether the drugs remain effective in pregnancy or are harmful to the baby, whether normal delivery is safe and whether breast-feeding is safe while on Crohn's drugs? This chapter aims to answer these questions and more, helping to make this period of your life as simple and exciting as it can be!

Crohn's disease from the medics

There has been a good deal of research trying to answer the questions highlighted above. No one can give advice that will definitely be correct for any individual's pregnancy and a careful discussion between the patient, her partner, her gastroenterologist and her obstetrician is the best way to assess risk in each case. Nevertheless, we have tried to produce some information here to help guide this discussion and help answer the important questions when considering pregnancy. Most of the evidence used to provide this information is based on expert/consensus opinion and data from modest, rather than powerful trials. Since Crohn's disease is often present in a person's reproductive years, these issues are very commonly discussed and considered, so your gastroenterologist will be experienced in giving advice relating to pregnancy, childbirth and breast-feeding.

Will I be able to get pregnant?

Women with inactive Crohn's disease have the same fertility rates as women in the general population. It is possible for Crohn's disease, due to inflammation or after surgery, to cause scarring in the pelvis, which can mean it is difficult for the egg to travel down the fallopian tubes and into the womb. Women with active Crohn's disease may have a slightly decreased fertility rate compared with other women. In spite of this, since fertility rates are similar overall between women with Crohn's and the rest of the population, particularly when their Crohn's is well controlled, it is usually a good idea to wait for a period of remission of Crohn's disease before trying to get pregnant. Men with Crohn's disease are no more likely to be infertile than other men, although Sulfasalazine is known to reduce fertility in men and this should be stopped two months before attempting conception.

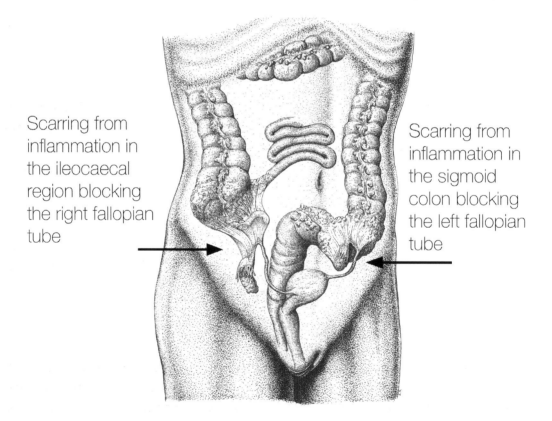

Scarring from inflammation in the ileocaecal region blocking the right fallopian tube

Scarring from inflammation in the sigmoid colon blocking the left fallopian tube

Figure 7. Demonstrating how scarring in the pelvis caused by inflammation in the terminal ileum and sigmoid colon might lead to 'pinching' of the fallopian tubes

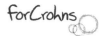

Will my Crohn's get worse during pregnancy?

Your Crohn's will probably be the same during your pregnancy as it was at the start of your pregnancy, although if you stop medication, there is a higher risk of a flare-up – just as there is if you stop your medication when you are not pregnant.

Will my child have Crohn's disease?

Children who have a parent with Crohn's disease have at least twice the risk of getting Crohn's disease or Ulcerative Colitis than the general population. This risk increases further if both parents have an inflammatory bowel disease. However the overall risk remains small and most children with a parent with Crohn's will not have the disease themselves.

How will my pregnancy go?

Women may worry that there is a higher risk of miscarriage, premature delivery, low birth weight or other problems associated with the pregnancy due to their Crohn's disease. Some studies have suggested that there is a slightly increased risk of caesarean section, premature delivery or low birth weight in Crohn's patients, but others have failed to confirm this or find an increased risk of any other problem associated with Crohn's itself. When added together in a powerful type of study called a meta-analysis, the evidence suggests that prematurity and low birth weight are more common in women with Crohn's than in the rest of the population. There is also some evidence that having active disease during pregnancy increases the risks, so it is usually recommended that women should avoid a flare of disease during pregnancy, and should try to conceive when the Crohn's is well controlled.

Should I change my diet during pregnancy?

Like any pregnant woman, it is important to ensure adequate nutrition and also to take supplements of Folic Acid. In Crohn's disease, particularly if active, sufferers may have worse nutrition than other women and also be less able to absorb Folic Acid, so increased dietary and Folic Acid supplements may be needed. This should be discussed with your gastroenterologist and obstetrician so your individual risk and needs can be assessed.

What about smoking and alcohol?

Smoking is bad for Crohn's disease, bad for pregnancy and bad for children to be around. At the risk of sounding preachy – smoking is a terrible idea in general, and even worse in a pregnant woman with Crohn's disease. Alcohol is also known to be harmful in pregnancy, and it is advised that all pregnant women avoid alcohol.

Are medications used in Crohn's disease dangerous during pregnancy?

Methotrexate and thalidomide should not be used during pregnancy by men or women and should be stopped long before a planned pregnancy, as they can be harmful to the unborn baby and cause birth defects. With the other drugs used in Crohn's disease, it is important to realise that there is little good scientific evidence about the risks of most drugs, for Crohn's or other diseases, and that the experience of experts is the best advice available. Most of the other drugs are thought to be basically quite safe because of the long-term experience of using these drugs in pregnancy, but it is difficult to know about long-term side-effects for certain. A careful discussion with your gastroenterologist and obstetrician to help understand the risks of continuing and stopping your normal drugs is important. While a concern about the risks of medication to your unborn baby is perfectly natural, a flare of disease may be harmful too and discussion with your doctors will help to balance these risks. The decision about whether to continue treatment depends on which drugs you take and your own personal circumstances.

Should I have a caesarean section?

Giving birth the normal way (vaginal delivery) is usually said to be better for mother and baby, and is the favoured way to deliver for women with inactive or mild IBD. However, one risk of vaginal delivery is damage to the anal sphincter (from a tear or episiotomy), which is the muscle you use to control your bowel and stop yourself from leaking. In most women, little if any damage occurs and the risk of difficulty in controlling your bowel is very low, but in Crohn's, healing of any tear may be very slow. Since women with Crohn's may have periods of diarrhoea at various points in their lives, control may be more difficult anyway, and any minor damage to the anal sphincter may cause more serious problems. However, most women will have no problems associated with a vaginal delivery. The decision about whether to have a caesarean section is therefore a personal one. The presence of a stoma does not prevent vaginal delivery either.

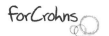
If, however, a woman has Crohn's disease around the anus such as an anal fistula or other active Crohn's disease in the area, a caesarean section is advised to avoid worsening of these problems and the risk of difficulty in controlling the bowel if any injury to the sphincter were to occur. This is an issue to discuss carefully with your gastroenterologist and obstetrician.

Is breast-feeding safe while taking my Crohn's medication?

Some drugs, after being absorbed by the mother, can be found in breast milk, which means the baby may also receive a dose of the drug she has taken. Some drugs are not found in breast milk at all, whereas others are found in large quantities. If taking steroids by oral tablet, it is sensible to wait at least four hours after taking the tablet before breast-feeding. Infliximab and adalimumab are also probably safe. Cyclosporine, methotrexate and some others are not safe during breast-feeding. Azathioprine is thought to be probably safe and can be used. If a woman stopped her treatment in order to breastfeed but developed a flare, she may then be too unwell to feed anyway and need surgery or additional medication. If planning to breastfeed, women should discuss this with their gastroenterologist and obstetrician before giving birth, so they can judge the risks and benefits of the different drugs they are taking.

Crohn's disease from the patients

The following part of the chapter looks at three patient stories from women who discuss their different experiences of pregnancy with Crohn's disease.

Wendy

Wendy is 49, married with one child and works as a writer. She was diagnosed with Crohn's when she was 19, has had many operations and would describe her Crohn's as 'moderate-severe'.

"I was 27 when I found I was pregnant for the second time. The first time had resulted in a miscarriage just three months earlier, followed by my surgeon – whom I both trusted and adored – telling me I probably shouldn't have a baby anyway; the risks were too great. It was unlikely my body would be able to nourish a child to full term and I would probably be hospitalised and on TPN for the last three months of my pregnancy. This time, I didn't care. I had considered it carefully, of course – I'd wondered if I had any right to have a child, when it was possible I would a) be unable to physically care for it properly and b) die before its 13th birthday. I don't know why I chose that particular age, it was completely arbitrary, but I convinced myself that any child I had would only have a mother until it was 12. This didn't come out of nowhere – my Crohn's was terrible back then, and my surgeon had predicted that I had two years to live about two years before my second pregnancy. I'd proved him wrong by then, obviously, but it was still a possibility that haunted me.

None of that mattered to me at this point though; I was pregnant and very happy about it. Rather romantically, we discovered the pregnancy the day after we got home from our honeymoon; newlyweds who would become parents in the next eight months or so – we'd never been so traditional in our lives!

Once my surgeon knew I was with child again, he didn't throw any more negatives at me, instead arranging for an early scan and telling me there were two ways pregnancy generally went in Crohn's patients – one was that the mother would be in good health right through the pregnancy and then get sick after the baby was born, and the other was that the pregnancy would be difficult and the mother would be fine once the baby was out. I was mostly the former. I felt pretty well, but we're talking comparatively here. I still took steroids (the risk to the baby was minor – a cleft palate seemed to be the scariest possibility) and instead of the regular blood transfusions I'd been having, I was prescribed iron injections, which were horrible. Not so bad going in, but painful and nasty for days afterwards, and just as they stopped hurting, it was time for the next one. The pain would radiate from the point of injection in a buttock, up the back and down the legs; it wasn't nice, but it was bearable and hey – at least it wasn't Crohn's.

The next thing that happened was they thought our baby might have *Down's syndrome* [1] – they saw water on the kidney, which often means a congenital disorder; that particular congenital disorder, in fact. I couldn't have an amnio, which would have told us for sure, because of all the surgery I'd had, and in those days there were no other ways of telling, so I just had regular scans once a month.

Oh, and they told us our baby was a boy, because that was a good thing – the water on the kidney meant Down's in girls far more often than boys. So we got excited about that, we chose a name and decided there was nothing we could do to change things, so we continued to celebrate being

> **1. Phil (surgeon) says:**
> This is not associated with Crohn's disease but is screened for in every pregnancy.

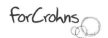

pregnant, between iron injections and monthly scans. At about the six-month scan, the radiographer told us he was pretty sure our little boy was going to be fine, but that if we ever quoted him, he would deny it. We loved him for that.

I was just about eight months pregnant – not having had to be hospitalised, or on TPN, or any of those other scary things – when my waters broke in the early hours of the morning. Waters always break in the early hours of the morning it seems. I have never heard of anybody having it happen just after lunch on a Saturday, when it would be convenient for everybody concerned. We dashed to the hospital and it felt so weird being there – being in the hospital where I'd had so many surgeries and this time, instead of leaving with less intestine than I'd had going in, I was going to be taking a real, live baby with me when I was discharged.

There were a few ups and downs. The first midwife I got was so useless, she couldn't even put the monitor around my belly properly, so I made my husband complain about her and get me a new one; the labour took a while to get started and eventually they induced me, but mostly it was fine. I realised that contractions felt pretty much exactly the same as the pain of an acute Crohn's attack and decided I didn't want any more of them thank you, so I had an epidural. After many hours of sleeping and talking, and a few less-than-enjoyable sessions where the lovely new midwife stuck her arm up inside me all the way to her elbow (at least, that's what it felt like), it was time to push, and I did. Suddenly our tiny little boy slithered out of me and my husband said, "Oh my god, Wendy, he's here". And he was fine, of course; not Down's, just our perfect, little bit small, little bit premature boy. They suctioned his lungs, then put him under *a grill thing* [2] to warm him up and he was gone. Leaving us, new parents, not quite able to comprehend what had just happened.

Later that night, they brought him to me, crying. Nobody could calm him down; they said he wanted me. His mummy. He was a funny-looking little thing. He prettied up in a couple of days, but you know how you wonder if you'd know if you had an ugly kid? Well, I knew. For those first 24 hours, he looked pretty damn weird, but I still loved him. And I held him and marvelled at his fingers and toes, and the fact that he'd come out of my tummy. That previously cursed place, full of ulceration and nastiness (not the uterus, I know, but the general area) had produced this little piece of total perfection. This little, tiny boy who stopped crying

2. Phil (Surgeon) says:
This is called a resuscitatire. Babies are often cold when they are born and midwives tend to rub them with a towel to dry and warm them, put them under the heat lamp in the resuscitatire and ultimately give them to their mother who warms them skin to skin on their chest.

when he was in his mother's arms. My arms. And I promised him I'd do my best never to leave him.

Luckily, I didn't remember my prediction of not making it past his 12th birthday until the night before he turned 13, so my neurosis on that point was mercifully limited. He's 19 now, and I'm still here and, thanks to ileostomy surgery in 2010, healthier than I've been in years. I think he's going to have to put up with me for a while yet."

Cassie

Cassie is 31, married with one child and works as a chemotherapy nurse. She was diagnosed with Crohn's when she was 14 and has had three operations. She describes her Crohn's as 'moderate' in terms of severity.

"So in January 2008, I was able to share the wonderful news with my family that I was pregnant. I had done some research on pregnancy and Crohn's, and everything stated that people in remission didn't experience any problems with pregnancy. I'd had a mild flare at Christmas (always at Christmas time!) but thought nothing of it, putting it down to overdoing it with party food. I loved being pregnant; it is the most amazing feeling in the world. The only problem I had was the morning sickness…which wasn't morning sickness; it was morning, noon and night sickness! I lost weight in the first few months, but the midwives assured me it was normal. They arranged for me to see a GI consultant, and I agreed as I hadn't seen my own consultant in a while. When I described to him how I'd been, he looked concerned and said I should start back on meds when the pregnancy was done. I can remember feeling really taken aback; I was so well! All I had described were the things I couldn't eat and the fact that I got pain if I didn't stick to the low residue diet, but he had seen something that I couldn't; that this was the *rumblings of the Crohn's* [3]. I chose to ignore him and refused his request to be seen after the pregnancy, saying I'd see my own consultant. It was a mistake for me not to talk to my doctors prior to getting pregnant, and not to arrange to see him throughout. I can see this now, but at the time I thought I was well enough not to need it. I was naive to the amount of strain a pregnancy puts

3. Phil (Gastro) says: Pregnancy has so many effects on the body that it is important to have regular reviews by your gastroenterologists – even if you feel well!

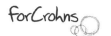

on your body. After giving birth, I was just over a stone lighter than before getting pregnant, but still it didn't twig that things were not right. To be honest, I was just happy that I didn't have lots of baby weight to lose.

In September that year, I gave birth to a gorgeous baby boy. Those early months were exhausting, but aren't they for everyone? Having a new baby is so exhilarating, you barely notice the tiredness. Only my fatigue seemed to be going beyond the norm. My diet was getting more limited and I suddenly realised that I was running to the loo way too much. My annual consultant appointment came around and he decided to restart some meds. I was upset because it meant stopping breast-feeding before I was ready (at about eight months), but I agreed. In hindsight, this was such a good decision. Ryan had been an unsettled baby, constantly wanting to feed and never putting on a great amount of weight. With the switch to formula, and weaning, he started to thrive. All I can imagine is that I didn't even have enough nutrients for myself, so didn't have enough to pass onto him. My guilt over not realising this sooner will be with me forever, but I can take comfort in the healthy wonderful young lad he is now!"

Sarah

Sarah is 30, married with one child and works as a respiratory therapist. She has had Crohn's disease for eight years and would describe it as 'mild' in terms of severity.

"I was diagnosed when I was 22. I'm now 30, and so far, the only surgery I've had to have is *my gall bladder removed* [4], so I consider myself more than lucky. They've put me on Remicade – my body didn't like it one bit, tried Humira, but had a bad reaction. So they offered me methotrexate, but I refused it, knowing it has the possibility of making having children a big fat no – and I knew my husband and I wanted kids together. I was left on Colazal, Protonix, Azasan and then my vitamins and supplements I take. I got married in November of 2011.

> **4. Phil (Surgeon) says:**
> This is not a Crohn's related operation. Gall stones are very common and can happen to anyone although some people with Crohn's may be at a slightly higher risk of getting gallstones because of a change in the way their bowel absorbs bile salts.

We took our honeymoon the following month in Missouri. We had a wonderful time and simply relaxed. All was amazing and my health was fantastic. Come January, I realise I'm not feeling 100 per cent, but attributed it to the Azasan as they had been adjusting my levels. I called my gastroenterologist, told them I was nauseated beyond belief and just worn out, so they sent me to have labs drawn. All was within normal limits. Then I realised... I was late, and every girl knows what I mean when I say I was late... I told my husband and we decided to wait a few more days to see if my body kicked in. It never did. So off to the chemist we go – and we buy the cheapest test there is – it was 50 per cent off. That sucker turned positive the minute it smelled my pee! We were ecstatic to say the least. Our families too! *The first thing we did was make an appointment with my obstetrician, then one with my gastroenterologist* [5]. My gastroenterologist had always told me, "when you get pregnant, let me know. I just want to be sure your health is great". Sounded like a deal to me and I was glad he was pretty protective, too. I saw the obstetrician, got a full bill of health from him. We told him I had Crohn's and he said, "not a problem, we can definitely handle it". Awesome, not only does he KNOW what Crohn's is, he knows it's controllable.

We saw our gastroenterologist, who was also very happy. He explained that I needed to watch my weight – if I didn't gain appropriately, I needed to call him as the Crohn's could be active and he might need to intervene. He then explained all my meds were fine to take, at which point I interrupted him and said, "Whoa, I already stopped the Azasan, I know it's a systemic med and it makes me nervous to take it while pregnant". He understood and said that being pregnant tends to be a magic cure for IBD, since your immune system is dropped to keep from hurting the baby. In a sense, pregnancy would *make me feel the best I have in a very long time* [6]. I honestly didn't expect to hear that, but yet I was relieved. I looked at my husband and I saw 20lbs come off his shoulders with that news. So, I stayed on Colazal, Protonix, and my supplements and vitamins. I've stayed as active as I can, and now being 39 weeks pregnant, I was just put on bed rest due to my blood pressure.

5. Phil (Gastro) says:
This is a very sensible approach. Discussing all the potential issues and seeking advice early on is likely to be very helpful in the long run.

6. Phil (Gastro) says:
It is true that pregnant Crohn's patients often feel better during pregnancy. However, the most important thing is to be well and have your Crohn's under as much control as possible – even if it requires medication. A happy Mum, means a happy baby!

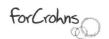

My Crohn's has stayed good. I saw my gastroenterologist again last month, who is still thrilled and said interestingly enough, he has another Crohn's patient due the exact same day I am. Will we both have our babies then? Who knows! He asked if I'm breast-feeding, I said yes, and he said to continue on my med regime as all are fine and won't hurt baby or be released into my milk. He said that our son's risk of getting Crohn's was very low (my husband is fortunate to not have IBD), and that made us both feel better. That was one of the main things that almost made me not want to have kids – the fear of passing this on to them – but breast-feeding, I hope, will help him not get Crohn's and *knowing there's no real genetic link* [7] makes me feel a world better. I saw my doctor again. He said I'll be protected another 90 days after delivery by my suppressed immune system and he feels 100 per cent sure that I'll do wonderfully. I'm very blessed, I know. I have an amazing team of physicians and a husband who loves and protects me and is there for me all the time. I hope my story shows there is hope; there is good that goes with this gnarly disease."

> **7. Phil (Surgeon) says:**
> There is certainly a genetic component to the cause of Crohn's disease but having Crohn's does not mean your child definitely will. However, if one parent has Crohn's or Ulcerative Colitis, any child is at a higher risk of developing the disease and if both parents have IBD the risk to the child is even greater.

Summary

As you can see, having Crohn's disease does not necessarily mean that you will not be able to have children – in fact, most women with Crohn's will be able to conceive, carry a child and have a normal delivery. It is important to speak to your gastroenterologist before you start trying to conceive, as some drugs may not be suitable to take during pregnancy and it is important to make sure that you are in the best health possible. If you are in remission, your fertility rates are around the same as the general population, and if the disease is active, your fertility is only slightly reduced. It is highly advisable to talk everything through with your medical team before trying to conceive to give you the best chance possible, and to ensure both you and your baby are in the best health possible.

Tips and suggestions

- **Before considering pregnancy, have a discussion with your gastroenterologist and obstetrician**
  This should include discussing whether the drugs you are on are safe in pregnancy and whether you should change any of your medications during your pregnancy, what kind of dietary supplements you might need to take and also whether a caesarean section is advisable (usually only if you have active disease around your anus). You should also discuss breastfeeding.

- **Aim to be in remission during pregnancy**
  This is preferable to falling pregnant during a flare of your Crohn's disease.

- **Listen to specific medical advice**
  For example, don't forget to take folic acid and stop smoking if you haven't already.

- **Keep an eye on your symptoms throughout**
  Monitor your weight throughout pregnancy and speak to your gastroenterologist if you have any symptoms that you are unsure about.

Being a child or young adult with Crohn's disease

For a child or young adult, being told that you have a serious condition needing investigation and complex treatments can be a frightening and lonely experience. One quarter of all patients with Crohn's disease develop the condition under the age of 16. Prior to diagnosis, many children have been unwell for a while, impacting on their schooling, with disturbing symptoms such as diarrhoea, pain, weight-loss and fatigue. Often, children will have a family relative or know someone who has Crohn's disease, and will be aware of the risk of surgery, and complications from the condition.

As a child who has just been diagnosed with Crohn's disease, you will have lots of questions about how it will affect your life, what tests and treatments you will need, whether you'll need an operation and so on. In this chapter, we try to answer these questions. Our specialist in treating bowel diseases such as Crohn's in children, has written the first section of this chapter and in it he describes how Crohn's affects children, who looks after them and what they can do to help. He also talks about the important issues that doctors consider when thinking about long-term diseases and their impact on children, such as growth, school and so on. Several children and young people have then written an account of their life with Crohn's as a child.

Crohn's Disease from the medics

Why children are different?

Compared to adults with Crohn's disease, the condition in children and young people is usually more severe and aggressive. The disease tends to present later to the doctors, as the symptoms are embarrassing to report to doctors and parents. Plus, while the condition is rare, there may be a delay before the diagnosis is recognised. Once seen by a *paediatric gastroenterologist* [1], parents are often relieved that "something is going to be done" – a sentiment that is not always shared by the affected child, as the next stage of investigations and treatments can generate fear and worry.

What happens next?

If the doctor considers that the child has Crohn's, care will be transferred to a paediatric gastroenterologist, often in a *specialist centre* [2]. These doctors have specific expertise in treating these complex conditions.

The affected child or adolescent will require an endoscopy (camera test, described in more detail in section 1) and although not painful, it is hard to tolerate without an anaesthetic or sedation. The endoscopy is likely to define the distribution of the Crohn's, which means it shows us how much of the bowel and which bits are affected, and how badly. This influences the choice of treatment. The endoscopy into the bottom (colonoscopy) needs to pass around a clean bowel, so medicines are given the day before the procedure, which cause diarrhoea. Such procedures may generate fear in a child and their family. Blood tests and special scans of the abdomen will take place around the time of the endoscopy.

Options for treatment in children

Crohn's in children needs a different approach to adults. *Steroid therapy* [3] is often used as a first option in adults, but this is not the case in children. By the

> **1. Phil (Surgeon) says:**
> A paediatric gastroenterologist is a specialist doctor who is expert in finding and treating bowel diseases like Crohn's in children.

> **2. Phil (Surgeon) says:**
> Since these problems are very specialised and not very common, children with Crohn's tend to be looked after in a hospital that specialises in bowel diseases in children with expert doctors. This may mean travelling further to see them but the trip will be worth taking!

> **3. Phil (Surgeon) says:**
> Steroids are explained in detail in the Drugs chapter as are the other drugs mentioned below.

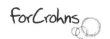

time Crohn's has been diagnosed in children, there is often poor nutrition, and sometimes poor bone health, with delay in puberty leaving children short for their age. Many of these factors prevent use of steroid medicines. For this reason, doctors recommend a special diet as the first choice for treatment – *"enteral nutrition"*. [4] If this is the preferred treatment option, the child might need to stop all solid foods and instead solely drink a specialised milky drink for up to eight weeks. In about 90 per cent of those who take enteral nutrition, the child will feel better within weeks of starting therapy and most children will catch up all the weight they lost, under dietetic supervision. The child and family can expect the disease to resolve temporarily on the enteral nutrition (which means their symptoms disappear and is called remission). For many children, this remission may last many months, or years.

On stopping the enteral nutrition diet, up to 60 per cent of children will relapse (meaning their symptoms return) within the first year, or develop symptoms again. While childhood Crohn's may be more aggressive than Crohn's in adult patients, the affected child is likely to be reassessed by endoscopy or scanning to see where the Crohn's has returned. Options at this point include starting *immune modifying medicines* [5] like azathioprine, mercaptopurine, or methotrexate which are effective in about 70 per cent of patients. Rarely, at this point, will the family might need to see a surgeon. For some, early surgery can *debulk the disease* [6] sufficiently to let the child grow.

> **4. Phil (Surgeon) says:**
> Enteral nutrition and other dietary treatments are explained in detail in the Diet chapter.

> **5. Phil (Surgeon) says:**
> Types of drugs discussed in more detail in the Drugs chapter.

> **6. Phil (Surgeon) says:**
> Surgery is usually not needed in children but occasionally it can be the best way to get the child into remission. Debulking the disease means removing affected areas so that the drugs used can be more effective and the symptoms or 'burden of the disease' are less. Surgery is discussed in detail in the Surgery chapter.

With a need to ensure the disease is in remission, or no longer active, doctors will want to start therapies one after the other until the child is better, both from symptoms and appearance at endoscopy. Children and adolescents may find they are on many different tablets, and supplements each day. Despite wanting to be free from symptoms, it is common that adolescent patients rebel against the medical advice and miss doses of tablets, keen to "just be like everyone else". This is obviously a bad idea, and the team would work with the family so everyone understands the role of each of the medicines. The most important thing is to make the disease resolve, even if this needs daily medicines.

Options for treatment include more novel therapies, such as biological therapies – within the first years of diagnosis. These include infliximab, which is given by a slow injection into a vein over a few hours. Alternatively, if necessary adalimumab will be prescribed which is a two-weekly injection. Both of these biological therapies carry risks, which will be discussed with the family.

Leaving active Crohn's disease in a child or adolescent is not acceptable, and every effort will be made to enable healing, to allow growth through puberty.

Impact of Crohn's on schooling

With ill health, investigations, treatments and appointments all happening at a critical time in adolescence and schooling, it may be hard to avoid impacting on education. Doctors are aware of this and will organise tests and appointments with the least disruption. However, undertreating the Crohn's can have detrimental long-term implications, and the symptoms of active disease will also affect school attendance – for example diarrhoea and pain might prevent children attending exams. In the first few weeks of treatment, children may not have the energy to compete in school games but as their health improves, within days or weeks, they should be strong enough to attend full-time education.

Impact of Crohn's on growth

This is the single most important issue that separates adolescent Crohn's disease from adult disease. Active Crohn's disease prevents growth, reduces appetite and nutrition and also has a detrimental effect on the state of bones. This culminates in delayed puberty, which makes the affected children shorter than their friends.

Effective Crohn's management can reverse these growth issues. Children can catch up on their puberty and growth, and their final height should not be affected by the disease. With growth threatened by Crohn's disease, paediatricians are less likely to offer a course of steroids as a treatment option. Many patients with Crohn's disease will see a paediatric endocrinologist, a specialist doctor who helps by assessing hormones and sometimes using hormone treatments to improve a child's passage through puberty and improve growth.

Adolescent issues with Crohn's disease

As explained above, Crohn's disease in adolescents comes with many challenges, but they can be overcome. Symptoms such as pain, diarrhoea, poor

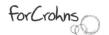

growth and lethargy should all improve on treatment. Investigations are tailored to adolescents by avoiding painful tests, organising for endoscopies to be performed under anaesthesia, and choosing radiology and X-rays that are safe to be repeated over time, to assess how well the Crohn's improves with treatment. Time off school is avoided. Treatment choices are selected for fast and lasting relief, even if this involves immune modifying medicines or surgery. Growth is assessed regularly and every effort is made to catch up on delayed puberty. The team includes psychologists and often patient groups to ensure the adolescent feels supported and not isolated by their disease.

Adolescents are encouraged to be part of all the investigation and treatment choices, including whether to have sedation or anaesthetic for endoscopy, and the role and timing of medicines. Adolescents must understand that smoking is particularly bad for Crohn's disease and is unwise at any time in adolescence. Many of the immune medicines used in Crohn's are dangerous for the unborn child. Therefore, families and adolescents will be approached to discuss birth control, or modifying drug choices to reduce the risk to an unborn infant.

Transition

By the age of 16-18 years, it will be time to move the adolescent from a paediatric-child clinic model into adult services. This process is called 'transition', where the paediatrician and the adult doctor will often work together over a period of months to ensure the family and adolescent gain confidence in the adult practice. Slowly over months, the family and adolescent move over to the adult or young persons' clinical services seamlessly.

Team members

Crohn's disease is such a complex disease that the child and family will meet many members of the gastroenterology team. This table on the next page describes the team members and their roles.

Team member	Role
Patient and family	Most important member of the team and support network. They are central to all choices about care and therapies.
Paediatric gastroenterologist	A paediatrician with expertise in investigating and treating children and adolescents up to 18 years of age with complex gut disease.
IBD nurse specialist	Works closely with the family and doctor, advising and preparing for procedures and organising treatments in hospital if necessary.
Dietitian	A specialist in nutrition who will take the lead for enteral nutrition and will support the patient with advice on the right diet.
Pharmacist	The patient is likely to need lots of different drugs. The doses and drug safety will be overseen by the pharmacist.
Paediatric nurses	Throughout the inpatient and clinic visits, these nurses will care for you and advise you each step of the way.
Radiologist	The doctor who uses scanners, and x-rays to assess the extent of the Crohn's disease.
Surgeon	Occasionally the Crohn's area needs to be removed, or tidied up to relieve symptoms or prevent complications. These skilled doctors know how to do this safely without pain and sometimes with only tiny scars.
Anaesthetist	Doctor who ensures all your tests are safe and pain-free.

Figure 8. Team members

Support for children and adolescents with Crohn's

Many children and their families find the best support is found from other families they meet on the inpatient ward or in clinic. Meeting other families who are living easily with Crohn's offers reassurance and can be a useful source of advice.

7. Contact details for these organisations can be found in the Links section at the end of the book.

Support is also available from the hospital that cares for the child – the staff are specifically trained to support and advise families with diseases like Crohn's. Useful websites with pamphlets suitable for children include *Crohn's and Colitis UK (formerly NACC) and CICRA* [7].

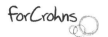

Crohn's disease from the patients

The following stories are written by young people who explain how Crohn's has affected their life, and their tips and strategies for managing the condition.

Paige

Paige is 16 and was diagnosed with Crohn's disease when she was nine. She would currently describe her Crohn's as 'mild'. In this story, she talks about her experience of living with Crohn's and the different tests that she had while in hospital.

"Being a baby who would projectile vomit most food that went past my throat, *it was no surprise that nine years later, I would be diagnosed with Crohn's disease* [8].

My dad has Crohn's, and I had often wondered what it would be like if I had it. What if I grow up to be like my dad? Would I have to go to the toilet for two hours in the morning before I even left my house?

I had just turned nine at the start of year four. I had this odd rash on my tummy that resembled

> **8. Phil (Surgeon) says:**
> Although Paige associates these things, vomiting in babies is very common and does not predict Crohn's disease in the future. However a family member with the disease does make someone more likely to have Crohn's.

chicken pox. I had had this horrible itching disease when I was about four, so it was highly unlikely that this was the pox. It baffled everyone and the doctors put it down to a virus. Then I began being sick in the middle of the night. It would wake me up suddenly, I'd throw up in my bed, mum and dad would change my sheets, then I'd go back to sleep. I'd stay off school the next day, then go back and I'd feel fine. This would happen probably about twice a month and each time the doctor would say it's food poisoning or a virus, and then he talked about Irritable Bowel Syndrome brought on by stress. My mum and dad were not convinced, but I had blood test after blood test, and nothing appeared abnormal. By this point, I had been sick on and off for about six months, I had lost a lot of weight and missed many days of school. My mum and dad had discussed Crohn's in the family to the doctor (my dad's sister also has Crohn's), but he had failed to see the signs! The doctor reassured us that there was nothing wrong with me. Until one night, when

I was so sick, it was clear that there was something seriously wrong and we needed to find out what. My mum and dad didn't think it was Crohn's, as my dad had never been sick; he had always suffered with stomach cramps and long periods spent in the toilet, but they knew something wasn't right. My doctor finally referred me to a specialist.

In the summer of 2004, on a Wednesday, I went to meet my specialist. I walked into his office at the Portland Hospital with my mum and dad, and as soon as he saw me, he was sure that I had Crohn's disease – something about my eyes looking sallow and my hair lacklustre. He asked me many questions before explaining to me that I would need an endoscopy. And that was the start… the next day I went into hospital.

> **9. Phil (Gastro) says:**
> We call this bowel preparation – it prepares and cleans the bowel for the colonoscopy by emptying it of all the faeces that are there. Many people find it more unpleasant than the colonoscopy itself, but it is very important as without it the colonoscopy cannot be performed.

To prepare for my endoscopy, I had to take the laxatives – drinking a mixture of something that tasted like flat lemonade (doesn't sound that bad, but trust me, it was!), and taking lots of tablets. *Let's just say this potent concoction caused me to spend the rest of the evening on the toilet!* [9] When morning came, I went down to theatre and my specialist confirmed what he had suspected.

So, at least we knew what we were dealing with. For the next eight weeks, I was to live on a liquid-only diet. I had to drink this horrible mixture called Modulen. My specialist explained to me that my tummy was full of little cuts and grazes (ulcers), and this soft 'milky' drink would give my tummy a rest so that these horrible sores could heal. My dad tried to convince me that it was chocolate milkshake and all my friends would be jealous of me! I'm not going to lie, it was the most vile thing I have ever had to drink! I refused to take it. Every time I'd take a sip, I'd heave! It wasn't until my specialist said that if I didn't take it, it would be need to be fed to me through a tube up my nose and down my throat, that I tried my hardest to down these shakes. We tried everything to make the process a little better. We would cover the cup (so I couldn't see it) and put a straw in it (so I couldn't smell it), and it did get better.

It was about a week before I agreed to go back to school after starting the Modulen diet, and without fail, my best friend Georgia and I would go to the school nurse to have my shakes. At the beginning, I would make her stand and hold my nose while I downed it using a straw, but as I got more used to it, I could drink it with her just standing and watching me. After that, she would go off to eat her lunch and I would watch the rest of the school enjoying their lunch (although I can't imagine the school food was worse than the Modulen). As if drinking it

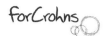

wasn't bad enough, one day the school nurse put one in the freezer by accident! Of course I had to drink it, but this time I had to eat it off of a spoon! After I had been a 'good girl' and drunk my shakes, I was allowed to have a boiled sweet – it was the only solid food that would pass my mouth for eight weeks.

The day finally came when I could eat again, but I had to be weaned very carefully, like a baby. My body had to get used to digesting food again. The first day I had chicken, and it was the best chicken I had ever tasted! It was dry and had no flavour, but it was a solid piece of food! Gradually, every day we introduced a little more. Every now and again I would be sick, but I slowly got back to normal.

From then on, my life started to become more normal – well, as normal as it was ever going to be for me. I still take a cocktail of drugs, and am still monitored very regularly. I know I have to be careful, watch my diet and not take my health for granted!

Having Crohn's as a child brought its difficulties, but thanks to the amazing support from my family and friends, I was able to get through the hard times."

Tanya

Tanya is 17 years old and studying for her GCSEs. She was diagnosed with Crohn's when she was eight years old and has had one operation. Tanya discusses her diagnosis experience and how Crohn's has affected her time at school.

"I was eight years old when I got diagnosed. I had just started a new school – a completely different one to my best friends. Being shy like me, I'm guessing the fear, stress and thought of being alone and friendless triggered my Crohn's. The first signs and symptoms were spots; I had *spots all over my arms and legs* [10]. My mum decided to take me to my local GP, who initially thought it was "flea bites" – this makes me laugh now, if only! At the same time, I was suffering from constant diarrhoea and I was slowly disappearing, but constantly being turned away from the doctors. Everything changed one morning. I woke up and my memory was blank, funny how I can remember it so clearly now; I couldn't remember anything – my brother's

> **10. Phil (Surgeon) says:**
> There are several skin rashes which are associated with the inflammatory bowel diseases including this one which was probably Erythema Nodosum. It is related to the activity of the patient's Crohn's and gets better on its own when the Crohn's flare settles.

name, how to work a tap, nothing. Later that day, after going to A&E, I was given my own room on a children's ward. I didn't mind it – every nurse was nice and my mum was there during the day (plus I've always known I wanted to be a nurse when I grow up, so it was rather interesting). It was the nights and the mornings I found most hard, waking up early and having to wait for my mum to visit always felt like forever, but looking back recently, it made me grow up and has done me good. We have to get used to it at some point! So after all the usual tests, they still didn't know what was wrong, so I was transferred to another hospital for my *first of many scopes* [11]. This is when I met my consultant who diagnosed me, put me on steroids and my meds – and I was perfectly fine for the next eight years with the usual scope here and there (bowel prep – eurghhhhh;)).

School is great. Of course I'm always worried about big changes, but I have my great friends for support; some new ones and some old friends from before my diagnosis. They all know how to make me happy. None of them fully understand Crohn's, but I don't expect them to. To be honest, I wouldn't want them to – it's rather embarrassing, however, we do occasionally joke about it. Recently I found out how much my friends meant to me, as the stress of my upcoming GCSEs and my great granddad passing away resulted in my Crohn's taking a battering! I was hospitalised for a few days and placed on the Modulen diet. With further tests, they decided this was not the right treatment and the next day I was transferred to another hospital –

awaiting emergency surgery to *remove my terminal ileum* [12] and appendix. It was there that I was first placed on an *adult ward* [13]. It was a hard experience to deal with as it's completely different to the children's ward I'm used to, however I met a lovely lady who also had Crohn's and we still talk now! Not only this, but my face

> **11. Phil (Surgeon) says:**
> Colonoscopy, a very good way of examining the large bowel (colon) and end of the small bowel (terminal ileum) where Crohn's is most often found. Colonoscopy is discussed in more detail in the Diagnosis chapter.

> **12. Phil (Surgeon) says:**
> This is quite a common type of operation for people with Crohn's disease to have. It is discussed in more detail in the Surgery chapter.

> **13. Phil (Gastro) says:**
> Over the age of 16, patients can no longer be looked after on the children's ward in the UK. This can be a strange experience for young people who are used to one kind of care and find themselves in a different environment. In preparation of moving from paediatric care to adult care, bigger hospitals run 'transition clinics' to prepare patients for this change.

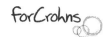

lit up when my friends came all the way to visit me. I will honestly never forget that day in January. Surgery went well and so far I feel OK since.

Having spent eight years with Crohn's – that's half my life now (weird) – I'm still learning! I used to be scared about the future, when it comes to relationships, work etc. but as it gets closer, I don't feel the need to be scared. I've got friends who are boys and they've reassured me there's no need to worry; I'm just a normal girl. I've also met people older than me who have been through it all and are now great friends, which is a great reassurance. And when it comes to work, I'm currently working hard for my GCSEs in order to do A levels that will get me into university to study children's nursing! I know it's hard work, but I'm determined! So when it comes to the future, I'm not scared – nowhere near! To be honest, I reckon Crohn's should be more scared than me!;)"

Alisha

Alisha is 15 years old and was diagnosed with Crohn's when she was eight. She has had 3 operations and would describe her Crohn's as 'severe'. Here she tells the story of her life so far living with the disease.

"I was born two weeks late and weighed 7lbs 12oz. When I was young, my mum said I was always a sickie baby and always had a sore bum. As I was growing up, no one would have ever thought I had Crohn's and Colitis because I was happy and never moaned. Between the age of two and five all that was a bother was my sore bum, but then my lips and gums started becoming sore. My *lips started to crack* [14] and then they split in the middle and I had to have them stitched up. My gums were becoming really sore and red, so I wasn't able to brush my teeth for a while. Eventually it was the dentist who knew what it was, *because of the lips and bum* [15].

14. Phil (Gastro):
Crohn's disease can present like this as a child with cracks in the lips – called angular stomatitis. Swollen, painful, ulcerated gums may be a condition called oro-facial granulomatosis (OFG) which dentists may recognise and then refer to a gastroenterologist.

15. Phil (Surgeon) says:
Crohn's disease, unlike Ulcerative Colitis, can affect any part of the gastrointestinal tract and quite often affects the anus or mouth. They become inflamed, sore and red which can be very unpleasant.

In year five, I started getting more poorly, and had to go into hospital for a *TPN line* [16] to be fitted to help me put a bit more weight on – I only weighed about two and a bit stone. I then got a bit better but had to go home on my first feeding tube. The special feed was called Alicalm and with that, there was no eating for six weeks – all I was allowed was water, Sprite and Polos. Having the *feeding tube* [17] was OK, but the worst thing about it was having it put in, as it's really uncomfortable but I had to either have the tube or drink it.

I started to get better. In year six, I was on a lot of medication, like azathioprine, steroids, iron, sodium and many more. I must have taken about 12 tablets a day – I hated taking tablets and medication but it made me better. I had a really bad belly near the end of year six, and I started stressing about going to high school which made me really poorly. I was worried what people might think of me because of how small and pale I was, and how swollen my lips always were. My family didn't want me to be sad and sit around all day doing nothing, they wanted me to go back to the old Alisha – who was always out playing till six o'clock and could stay up late at sleepovers instead of going to bed at eight.

In year seven, I fell really ill because of the stress about what people thought and worrying about whether people were calling me a 'midget' because of my size and 'fish lips' because of how swollen they were. Sometimes I just wanted to tell everybody about my condition so they knew why I was so small and had such big lips, but was afraid of what people might think – maybe it would make things worse.

I was so stressed out that I only went to school for two months, and then had to have an operation, which was for a stoma to be fitted. It was my only option, otherwise the abscess would have burst and I could have died. I had a while off school to recover, then eventually I went back and my friends were really supportive when I told them about it. They weren't that shocked because we had talked about it before, and we all knew that one day I would have to have

16. Phil (Surgeon) says:
TPN is total parenteral nutrition which means a complete supply of all the nutrients your body needs straight into the vein. This allows the bowel to rest whilst still providing you with nutrition. The line is a plastic tube placed into the vein in the neck which is done under local anaesthetic and is a bit uncomfortable when it goes in but doesn't hurt at all once it is in place.

17. Phil (Surgeon) says:
The feeding tube is a plastic tube that goes through the nose and down into the stomach. As Alisha says, putting it down is not very nice but once it's there it's not too uncomfortable and the feeding tubes are very narrow indeed.

166

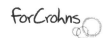

one. A week later, this other girl who knew about it told me her nanna had just had one fitted – her nan didn't like having one, but I reassured her that she'd get used to it. But after two weeks at school, my intestines got stuck together, which was really painful. I couldn't walk straight or eat but we didn't know what it was until I had an ultrasound scan. This was all after just two weeks of being in year eight, but I had already started to feel a lot more confident about myself.

> **18. Phil (Surgeon) says:**
> A fistula is a tunnel of infection, in this case from the bowel to the skin. Crohn's causes fistulas to the skin, around the anus or in between the bowel and other organs. Not everyone gets fistulas but they can be difficult to deal with when they appear.

Not long after, a big *fistula* [18] appeared next to my stoma, so I wasn't allowed to eat or drink until they got it sorted. They thought they would have to take my whole bowel away, but then decided just to leave it to heal on its own.

I've not been back to school since year eight. At the beginning of year nine, I went back into hospital with two more fistulas, but I was only in for six weeks this time. The only option was to have the same operation, but on the other side of my tummy. I went home a week after the operation, where I am now, and I'm feeling better than ever. I have grown a lot and put weight on. It was a really tough time. I had my ups and downs but who wouldn't, being stuck in hospital? It's been an experience that I will never forget, and hope it has helped you, whoever is reading this.

I couldn't have got through it without my friends and family there every step of the way. My family never let me down, they all helped with looking after me. My mum would stay at the hospital most of the week, then at the weekend maybe a friend would stay, or my stepdad, nan or aunt, or even my next-door neighbour. We all always had a fab time whatever we did. Sometimes we would just sit and talk, or watch a film – always scary movies, they're the best. I would always make the nurses jump on Halloween:). The nurses helped me a lot, too. At the end, one of them gave me £5 for a takeaway because of how long I hadn't eaten for. Of course I spent it as soon as I could!

My friends were really helpful. If I needed anything, they would get it if they could. I would ask if they could update me on all the gossip at school, school work etc. If there was an important piece of homework, they would always bring it up when they could. It was difficult because we all live in Doncaster and I was staying in Sheffield Children's Hospital – but we still kept in touch. I would ring them every day, text morning, noon and night.

Crohn's has had a huge effect on my life. I've not been able to go to friends and sleep over because of the tiredness and I've lost out on a lot of important school years. It's had an effect on my family's life too, but I am so much better now. With the stoma, there is no more rushing to the toilet or not having an appetite. I now weigh 33kg. Going from 23kg to 33kg is a lot, so my mum bought me a whole new wardrobe. I used to wear years 8-9 sized clothes, but now I'm an adult size six – though I still need a size 13-14 in trousers because I'm still not the tallest person (I'm 4ft 8inchs).

I am currently very busy organising three fundraising events and have just chosen my options for year 10, getting ready for my life ahead. The doctors have also said that when I've got through my GCSEs, I can have the stoma reversed if I want. My mum would say I'm a lot more mature for my age because of what I've been through, but I'm still Alisha and no one can take that from me. But I must admit, I wouldn't be me without Crohn's – and my life would probably have been boring without it.

You can get through it every step of the way. Don't give up, keep fighting and together we can beat Crohn's:)"

Adam

Adam is 26 years old and was diagnosed with Crohn's when he was 11. Adam is currently a musician and would describe his Crohn's disease as alternating between 'severe' and 'stable'. He recalls his experience with Crohn's throughout school and university.

"My Crohn's story began many years before I was even aware that I had Crohn's disease. Although I was diagnosed at 11, I don't remember a time going through primary school when I was not going to the medical room, complaining of an upset stomach of some kind. It must have been such a regular occurrence that I am told I even invented my own name for it – the 'tummy headache'. After persistent tummy complaints, my mother eventually insisted that my doctor refer me to a gastro specialist. After visits to doctors at various hospitals in London, and after a few misdiagnoses, I was eventually diagnosed with Crohn's disease. At the time, I was probably not quite mature enough to understand the implication of this diagnosis. At the same time, I had grown up always having these health issues, so I had learnt to deal with it pragmatically.

My Crohn's played a big part in my life at secondary school. My time there was spent mostly with active Crohn's, with periods of remission in between. It

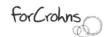

reared its ugly head at the *most difficult of times* [19] – during my GCSEs and A Levels. The first time my Crohn's severely affected my school life was just after I turned 13. I was going through a very stressful time at home due to divorcing parents, and about a month after my birthday, I ended up in hospital for a few weeks. This was very difficult because I was very conscious of keeping up with things at school, and so I knew I was going to fall behind with many activities, not just academic.

The solution the doctor proposed was an *elemental diet* [20], where you give up eating for a period of time, and replace it with a special formulated drink containing all the necessary nutrition of a stable diet. Now, these were the days when they did not have a variety of flavoured protein drinks – I just had powder that came in a big metal tin, which when mixed with water, formed a milkshake-like drink. This was such a huge thing for me, as I loved my food, and I had been told that I needed to give it up for eight weeks. I even remember the last meal I had the evening before I started it. I had a margarita pizza, and saved a little bit to put in the freezer, to be defrosted once my 'detox' had been completed. This was just one aspect of my problem. The other thing playing on my mind was wondering how people at school would react to me coming into the canteen and, instead of eating the moderately tasty school dinners, taking a thermos flask out of my bag, and tucking into a liquid lunch of 'CT3211'. This was the code name for the powder, as it was on trial and didn't even have a real name, so it stuck with me for some obscure reason. I like to think that it was my quirky sense of humour that allowed me to think of my diet as a code of letters and numbers. I eventually got through this period of relapse, and back into remission.

Sixth form was another difficult time, as I had another flare-up. Although on this occasion I didn't end up in hospital as an inpatient, I did *miss a significant amount of school* [21]. This fuelled the vicious cycle of stress due to missing school and worrying about exams, which in turn exacerbated my condition. It came to a point when I was so worried about how my A Levels and subsequent future would be affected, that I took it upon

> **19. Phil (Surgeon) says:**
> This is a common story and there is a great deal of research which suggests that Crohn's flares and periods of life stress are often associated with each other.

> **20. Phil (Surgeon) says:**
> This diet and similar therapies are discussed in the Diet chapter.

> **21. Lucy (IBD Nurse):**
> If Crohn's disease is affecting your ability to attend school or college or university, extra support is available. Please let your IBD nurse or gastroenterologist know.

myself to contact teachers to email work to me, and then I could email them if I felt I needed particular help. Luckily I got myself well enough to take the exams. I also qualified for 'special consideration' when it came to my results, and I ended up doing really well considering the circumstances. I had lots of willing and helpful teachers, but my family were the real stars. Combined, I had experts in maths and sciences. I also got tutors for other things. My A Levels were in maths, physics, music and Spanish. I got the results I needed to go to music college in Leeds to study drums on an undergraduate performance degree course, but the active disease was to make another, more profound appearance.

During the summer after I finished my A Levels, I became very ill again. This time, the steroids and other drugs did not seem to work. I was so desperate to be well enough to go to music college, so I suggested I try the elemental diet again. I also went all gung ho with alternative therapies. I saw a medical herbalist, a hypnotist, and an acupuncturist. I had about a week or so before I was due to leave for uni, and things were looking very bleak. I had worked so hard through my A Levels, and probably missed about half of the school time in total, so I was praying that it would be worth the struggle. In the week that followed, I made such a huge amount of progress – I went from being in constant pain and needing to rest, to being a spritely 18 year old, ready to take on life as a student musician. I was so excited to be going through with it that arriving at my halls of residence with three crates of drinks for my elemental diet seemed rather insignificant. I also ended up with four flat mates who were all really easy-going and chilled out (they were all musicians – it was inevitable). I would continue to have minor flare-ups during my three years at college, but it was all managed with medication to a point that I could still carry on doing what I was doing."

Terry

Terry is 20 and works part-time as a sales assistant in retail. Terry was diagnosed with Crohn's when he was 11 and has had two operations. He would describe his Crohn's as being 'severe'. This is Terry's account of his life with Crohn's.

"You will never do anything in this world without courage. It is the greatest quality of the mind next to honour" – **Aristotle.**

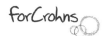

"So let's start at the beginning. From the very young and innocent age of five I remember having a good appetite. I was extremely active too; I would swim four times a week, later on doing martial arts up to three times a week and playing football in my back garden. I soon joined a team. Apart from being slightly shorter than my peers, there wasn't anything going on to suggest there was a devastating, life-changing disease growing or about to appear inside of me. I always seemed to have lots of diarrhoea attacks that lasted for days, even weeks, causing me to be very skinny despite my active lifestyle. I had several appointments with doctors through the years of four to about nine, where they kept saying "It's just a bug, it'll be gone in a few days" so I wouldn't be allowed anything 'rich', just dry bland foods like toasts and dry biscuits – and sure enough, the symptoms were gone. Three months later, we'd go through the same process again; we just thought I was unlucky.

Then my final year of primary school came and there would be times when suddenly I stopped walking and couldn't move (I was having stomach pain). I didn't understand it, neither did mum, she thought I was faking. This would happen more and more. People from outside my family began to see it. While at martial arts kneeling down, I would have stomach pain and twist my torso against it to make it more comfortable or just simply make it go away. My teachers would ask if I was OK. "Sure" would always be my reply. This often happened during football, too. I would stop, sit on the ball and 'look all sad'. Sometimes when the sensation went, I would bounce right back up and carry on playing, but sometimes I just wanted to go back inside – I had lost my energy. It wasn't long before I became an 'indoors kid', though I would still do martial arts – that was vital for school as I was often picked on, looking defenceless on my own in the playground.

Once we had picked up on recurring symptoms, we went to the doctors and got several misdiagnoses; we were told I had Abdominal Migraine. I had some treatment for it; nothing special, just a pill or something, and it was 'OK' for a time. I was going to secondary school in a few months and the symptoms started again. This time, violent pain was a lot more evident and I knew I had something really bad. I thought I was going to die from one of these pains or I had stomach cancer (at nine or 10, that's not what you expect a kid to be thinking about). We continued going to the doctors who kept trying, and doing blood tests through the summer holidays and I was bracing myself for what was going to be a massive chapter in my life. Not only was I about to go to 'big school' and become more independent, but I was about to be given the massive bombshell that is Crohn's disease.

"What can't be cured must be endured" – *English proverbs*

It was the second day of secondary school, I knew two or three people from my previous school and everyone was very nervous. 15 minutes into the school day and the head of year seven came in and called my name. She pulled me outside my class and said "Terry, stay calm (I'm thinking "HOLY CRAP WHATS GOING ON?!") your mother is in reception. She is very worried because this morning she received a letter about you from the doctors who are concerned and need to see you urgently".

The doctor wanted to do another blood test and told me that my iron and vitamin C levels were low, so prescribed me some meds for that and told me to eat oranges. "Could I go back to school after my blood test please?" I asked. "No, you might go 'funny' afterwards, just come home and go to school tomorrow". I was very disappointed, but I carried on with eating my satsumas and took my iron medicine (which tasted like blood, very nasty). About three hours later, my Crohn's erupted. I'm not a screamer when it comes to pain, nor showing it or taking pain-killers, but those pains were like nothing I had ever felt before. They were so long, about 20 minutes each, and just felt like lava was passing through my bowels. I often describe my pains as acid on a sword. I was rolling around on my bed. I couldn't hide it from mother – she watched on in horror for 45 minutes. My mother consulted with our neighbour who said to ring NHS direct. They were clueless and sent out an ambulance. It arrived and I got up and tried to get in normally, but they shouted at me to walk slowly. I was puzzled because it was stomach pain – not a broken leg or back? I got in and they gave me oxygen. I pushed it away "I CAN BREATHE, MY STOMACH JUST REALLY HURTS YOU MORON!" (When in pain, I am prone to lash out verbally to anyone that remotely annoys me. This only came about since having Crohn's disease). We got to the hospital and they asked me lots of questions – same old, same old. They gave me some pain-relief which tasted really nice! I talked to numerous doctors and nurses, one of whom took a lot of interest in me – she sat me up, looked into my eyes, held my hands and rubbed my thumbs, she looked at them, then back into my eyes and said "there's something really wrong with you honey, we are going to find out what it is though". I really couldn't grasp what was going on, it was surreal, and even though at times it dragged, it happened so fast.

About 12am, I was approached by a nurse who apologised about how late it was, asking me the same questions. She was confident in her reply: "it's Crohn's or Coeliac Disease, we are going to have you in next week for a colonoscopy so

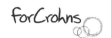

we can see inside you properly, and find out what it is". I didn't really know what to think about it all, I just wanted to go home and have a fry up.

The colonoscopy happened and I was eventually told "you have Crohn's disease... it's... incurable but..." I burst into tears. I couldn't deal with this. I was deemed 'unshakable' to this point. I didn't care what it was called, it was the word 'incurable' I focused on. I was told I would then undergo treatment right away. I wasn't allowed any food whatsoever – I was to be started on the 'wonderful' liquid diet that was Modulen IBD. A milkshake product that was designed to give

> **22. Phil (Surgeon) says:**
> This is a very understandable reaction but in fact being fit and strong will help you have the strength to recover when you're ill. It is unlikely that even a strenuous sport will cause you damage but if you've recently had surgery it is sensible to discuss when you can return to contact sports with your surgeon.

me all the nutrients I required that I wasn't having in order to put weight on. Absolutely disgusting. I was also on Pentasa tablets which were very big and not easy to swallow. It was a very difficult time; I had spent no time in school and wasn't looking at going back anytime soon. I was told by my doctor that I would most likely never go to university and therefore get a decent job. I had to be able to show I was taking the medication and it was working. *Mum forced me to quit martial arts* [22], afraid I was going to be hit in the stomach, which would make me bad, and the same with football. "You just don't know", she would keep saying. I was wrapped in cotton wool – mum's youngest had an incurable disease and there was nothing she could do. That's one thing with Crohn's, it's not just you that is battling it. Your closest family will too, and your friends will look after you.

I continued to have problems on and off during secondary school. It got to a stage where I had to go back onto Modulen again to keep my nutrients up. Later on that week, I had an emergency consultation in Bristol with a surgeon, as my barium showed I needed surgery. And so I was admitted, and nil by mouth, I was potentially having an operation within 24 hours – but no space opened, so it was going to be in two days' time (a Thursday). They told me everything they would do, what would happen after and how I would feel. I wasn't scared at all, I was never scared when facing positive action and I was also never scared until it was literally about to happen. To me 'taking away any infected bowel' seemed to be a brilliant idea – I'm a firm believer in removing the problem completely, rather than leaving things inside.

So Thursday came, and I was told it would be about 2pm that I would be wheeled down to 'OR' and have the operation. I started to become tense, it was happening. Time went so slow, minutes felt like hours. The worry in my mother's face was for all to see. I had to be the rock she needed. I had to show no pain. I had to be calm because no one else was. People wanted and expected me to break down in tears. I didn't believe in that. I gathered a great strong character from playing games based on legendary warriors and tactical thinkers set thousands of years ago – I felt their strengths seep into me.

Being in a children's hospital made the experience 'nicer'. The nurses are more friendly and courteous and there are no random old guys walking around with those backless gowns. Also, the nurses took to me very quickly. They could tell I was very grown up for my age and easier to talk to, I made no fuss despite how critical I was and how much attention I required.

A while after the operation, my Crohn's seemed dampened and I was on just azathioprine. I was active, I was social, and I even started enjoying sitting in the sun. Year 11 was the best year I had in secondary school, teachers couldn't praise me enough. I did well in all of my choices, getting a C average with a few Bs, too. The teachers couldn't believe it; they said if my illness was under control early on, there was no telling what I could have done. I was proud with what I did, and I didn't feel I had put that much effort in. In my eyes, I had done what was needed.

So after finishing secondary school in the spring of 2008, I was about to be more social and my condition was in a nice state of remission. In year 11, I had only missed seven days of school, a record! In the summer, I had my first actual girlfriend; it didn't feel like a year since my operation. A massive transformation, I was going to go into sixth form (otherwise known as college), to study drama and sport.

> **23. Phil (Surgeon) says:**
> Adalimumab (Humira) is a similar drug to Infliximab.

Things were going well. And my first half of the year went great and very quickly. Suddenly, I started getting symptoms again. BAM! Where did this come from, the Crohn's launching a surprise attack? We got it seen to, quickly. I was no longer under the Bristol people. I had now become 'adult age' and was able to have a gastro at my local hospital. He reacted very quickly, putting me on aggressive medication called 'Humira' [23]. I liked this doctor; he was quick, thorough and wanted me to be better. I remember not being too keen on injecting myself, as my mother is not a fan of needles. However soon after, for the first time since having Crohn's, I was able to look into the future, plan for it and attack it rather than waiting for the next phone call from the hospital for the next course of action with medication."

Terry went on to university, but had a further severe attack of Crohn's and left. He now works in retail and is planning the next phase of his life with renewed energy and his continuous positive attitude.

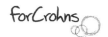

Courtney

Courtney is 13 years old and was diagnosed with Crohn's when she was eight. In this story, she talks of her experience, including having a colostomy bag.

"My name is Courtney and I am 13 years old. I was first told I had Crohn's when I was eight. At first, I was really scared because I did not know anything about the disease and I did not know what it was. We got *loads of information from the doctors* [24] and I got taken into hospital for a scope, which helps the doctors know what is going on inside. I have had many of these before. I have had NG tubes a lot, too. Then when I was 10, I got a colostomy bag fitted *and a button in my belly for this milk* [25] that makes you put weight on. I was scared of what my friends would think about me and I thought my life was over. But the colostomy bag didn't really change my life at all, I just have to be careful with what I do and if it leaks, I just have to make sure I have spare bags wherever I go. My friends don't really care about me having

24. Phil (Gastro) says:
This is one of the most important roles of the doctor making a new diagnosis and s/he will often involve an IBD specialist nurse in the discussion both to help but also to provide a contact the patient and their family can turn to for advice and support in the future.

25. Phil (Gastro) says:
The 'button in the belly' Courtney is referring to is a feeding tube which means that Courtney can be given drugs and nutrition directly into her stomach. It is called a PEG tube normally and can be inserted via an endoscopy procedure by a gastroenterologists or via x-ray guidance

it, they just see me as normal. I used to think that I was strange, compared to other people. At the beginning of the year, I had another operation where they removed some more of my bowel, but the operation did not go very well. It was a few weeks later that I realised that at the side of my stoma (colostomy), there was a very deep hole. They had to get me on the morning list the next day and I stayed in hospital for nearly four months.

Crohn's is a big part of my life now, and it has affected my confidence. I hardly ever do things that teenagers do – like climbing and stuff. I can't run about for that long, as I can get tired quickly. At school, I am off a lot. The biggest support in my life is probably my friends or my mum. I turn to my mum if I need help with my colostomy bag or if I feel unwell or just a bit down about my condition. My family help me every way they could when I was in hospital – visiting me as much as they could. The main thing that helps with my confidence is not to let my disease take over my life, as it is a part of me and I am who I am! My friends help me a lot with my confidence. They are always there for me when I need them. The main tip I can give is just get on with life and don't say you can't do something because of your condition."

Summary

It is understandably a difficult time for both the child and their parent when they are given the diagnosis of Crohn's disease. The strength that they have to gain from a young age and the knowledge they develop of the disease can be truly amazing. It is important for the child and their carers to understand the disease and to know the triggers that they may have. It is helpful for a child to recognise the warning signs of a flare-up from a young age, so when they leave children's care and are seen as an adult patient, it is not too much of a transition for them. This transition can be a worrying time, but the paediatric gastroenterologist will help the child and their family through the process. As you can see, our authors have been determined not to let Crohn's bring them down and they have been successful at school despite time off for surgery for example, gaining jobs or places at university and succeeding in them.

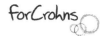

Tips and suggestions

- **Keep a food diary**
  Notice the foods that 'upset' your tummy, and stay away from them.

- **Listen to what your specialist suggests**
  Take the medication you are prescribed.

- **Speak to your teacher about having Crohn's**
  Let them know that you may need to rush off to the toilet during lessons.

- **Allow yourself more time to get ready in the mornings**
  Some days you will need the toilet more than others, so it is best to give yourself lots of time so you won't start stressing about being late.

- **Be active**
  This can sometimes take your mind off of the pain or stress you are going through.

- **Keep a social life**
  Get on with your life as best you can. Having other people around you can take your mind off Crohn's, or if it helps, speak to your family and friends about your worries.

- **Try not to get too stressed**
  This can irritate your Crohn's.

- **Stay strong, and remember you are not the only one going through this!**
  Join Crohn's charities and networks. This is a great way to meet people going through the same thing as you. Try to contact someone else who has Crohn's, as they know exactly what you are going through and you can help each other get through difficult times.

Psychological impact of Crohn's disease

Being diagnosed with Crohn's can have not only a physical effect, but a psychological one too. This is the case with any chronic disease, but perhaps particularly in the case of Crohn's (and similar diseases) when there is limited awareness and understanding amongst the general public, and the problems associated with the disease lead to embarrassment when discussed. We hope this chapter will help to give more understanding of these psychological difficulties; both through explanation from an expert (Dr Julian Stern) and individual stories from those with the condition.

Crohn's disease from the medics

Most cases of Crohn's disease begin before 30, with the illness often starting in young adulthood. 20-30 per cent of all patients with Crohn's disease are diagnosed before 20. There is then a second peak of new cases occurring between the ages of 60 and 80.

What is the psychological impact of this illness that often affects teens and young adults? And what can be offered to help patients with Crohn's cope better with the impact of their condition?

The teenage and early adult years are years of substantial emotional change and challenge. Adolescence is a time of developing independence. Sexual identity becomes established. There is an intense preoccupation with appearance

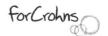

and change in body image, an exploration of the balance between intimacy and individuation, grappling with fears of merging on the one hand and isolation on the other.

Already, even without an illness like Crohn's disease, adolescence is a complicated time in our life.

So, in this time of emotional upheaval, when one might be moving away from home, starting work or college, be involved in exams or a first sexual relationship, and immensely preoccupied with one's body and body image – what is the impact when one's body starts misbehaving, breaking down from within – in the most delicate and private of areas: the bowels, rectum, and anus?

Research from around the world shows that around 1 in 4 patients with IBD (both Crohn's disease and ulcerative colitis) can probably be diagnosed as suffering – at some stage – from anxiety or depression, and about 1 in 2 patients have some features of anxiety or depression, but not severe enough to fulfil the conditions for a definite diagnosis.

These figures are in keeping with the rates of anxiety or depression in patients with other chronic illnesses like rheumatoid arthritis or diabetes.

Another study found a 14-16 per cent rate of depression in any one year of patients with IBD, and found that a full 40 per cent of such patients were on an antidepressant. Rates of psychological distress (depression) are higher in women, those without partners, in younger patients, those with greater pain and those with functional limitations.

One way of looking at these figures is to see that compared with the general population, patients with Crohn's are at greater than average risk of developing anxiety or depression. But which patients will go on to develop anxiety or depression? And an equally interesting question is what protects patients with Crohn's from all developing anxiety or depression?"

The illness can clearly lead certain patients to becoming depressed or anxious. Other psychological syndromes or symptoms associated with the illness can include:

- Phobias (e.g. needle phobia, fear of stomas, hospital phobia).

- Post Traumatic Stress Disorder (e.g. following particularly traumatic periods in hospital).

- Eating disorders (including the dangerous combination of Crohn's and anorexia, with both illnesses contributing to weight loss).

- Obsessive compulsive symptoms.

- Addictions to pain killers which can become habit-forming.

In addition, due to the complicated and intimate nature of the illness, the following developmental issues are frequently seen in practice:

- Anxieties to do with separation from one's family.

- Anxieties to do with establishing intimate relationships.

- Sexual anxieties.

- Body image anxieties.

What can be offered to help?

Not all patients with Crohn's disease require psychological support from a professional – many cope very well with support from a combination of family, friends, partners, and colleagues at work, as well as the support offered by professionals such as the GP, hospital doctors, IBD support nurse, dietitian, and stoma nurse (where relevant).

There is evidence from the literature that many patients benefit from psychological therapy, with regard to their mood and mental state, and in some cases with regard to the disease activity itself. This is not widely available in the UK, and provision of services, especially specialised services for patients with Crohn's, is patchy.

So, for those patients who feel that they DO require something extra, the options are as follows:

1. Voluntary sector organisations and charities

CCUK (Crohn's and Colitis UK) is a large and very well-known organisation that brings together people of all ages who have been diagnosed with IBD, their families and the health professionals involved in their care.

Amongst its many activities and resources, it provides Crohn's and Colitis Support (formerly NACC-in-Contact) which was established in 1989, in response to the many patients and relatives seeking confidential personal support in coping with ulcerative colitis or Crohn's disease. In addition to their group structure, they provide a range of activities that include:

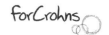

- Regular self-help or support group meetings

- Educational meetings with a speaker or panel of experts

Question and answer sessions

Other charities and patient support organisations offer a multitude of resources. One example being (amongst many others):

- IA – the ileostomy and internal pouch support group – an online support group for patients with ileostomies

2. NHS Help

While the psychological needs of many patients are satisfied by the organisations mentioned above, others will require more formal psychological support.

The first port of call often is the GP. S/he may be able to offer some support or counselling in the GP surgery, with a counsellor or primary care psychologist attached to the practice.

The GP may also suggest tablets – usually an anti-depressant. You should be aware of both the possible benefits of such tablets, and of their possible side-effects. They can, on occasion, lift your mood and reduce anxiety. However, they are not a magic solution to all the difficulties, and cannot sort out some of the more complex issues and anxieties raised by the disease.

In recent years, there has been an increase in the provision of primary care psychology services and your GP will know how to access this help.

If you are referred to this service, called IAPT "Improving Access to Psychological Therapies" or Primary Care Psychology, the first contact may be by telephone. Depending on the severity of your symptoms, you might be offered either face to face work with a therapist, or telephone contact, or be referred to self-help books in the library, or even to a computerised programme of CBT (computerised Cognitive Behavioural Therapy). Patients vary as to whether they find these methods helpful or acceptable.

If the IAPT/primary care service is not sufficient, you may be able to be referred to more specialised psychological resources, called secondary care psychology or psychotherapy services. These will be part of the provision of more specialised services, either as part of your local mental health provision, or in some cases, attached to the gastroenterology department in which you are being looked after.

These resources are scarce. The best known example is the St Mark's Hospital Psychological Medicine Unit, attached to St Mark's hospital in Harrow (London), which receives about 200 referrals per annum of patients with gastroenterological disorders also needing psychological assessment and/or treatment. Not all of these have Crohn's, but a significant proportion (about 30 per cent) do; and not all can be treated by this one unit. More resources are undoubtedly needed throughout the UK.

Currently, much of the psychological care of the Crohn's patient is held by the GP, the IBD nurse and the stoma nurse – all often excellent, but none specifically an expert on specialised psychological techniques.

Types of psychological therapy

Options for therapy depend very much on staff availability and mix.

Some patients are treated by focused work, focusing on their beliefs and behaviours (CBT), especially if there is a phobia, high degrees of panic and anxiety or obsessionality involved.

Some are best treated as part of their family or as a couple (couple or family therapy).

Some require longer-term therapy to try to help explore the roots of their problems, and how the disease interacts with their early years, their personality and their families of origin (psychoanalytic psychotherapy).

Others are helped by being in a group with other patients with the same illness (group therapy) or others suffering from other chronic illnesses. Alternatively, some feel they want to be in a group with no one who shares the same illness, so as not to feel too submerged in a Crohn's world.

EMDR (eye movement desensitization and reprocessing) is a treatment used to work with patients who are traumatised, and suffering from Post-Traumatic Stress Disorder. Not very available in the UK yet, it is recommended in the NICE (National Institute for Clinical Excellence) guidelines for PTSD.

Finally, there are increasing numbers of treatments using internet chat rooms, web-based forums etc. Some of these are being piloted by psychology and psychotherapy organisations, and may well prove to be a useful resource for patients with Crohn's disease.

3. Private options

If you have private medical insurance, or choose to go privately, it is possible that you will choose to go to a private practitioner for psychological help.

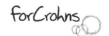

Always try to use a reputable organisation, and ask your GP or specialist for advice about whom to see.

There are professional organisations that require their members to work according to professional and ethical standards, and you could use these as a starting point.

For psychoanalytic psychotherapy, use a practitioner recommended by the BPC (British Psychoanalytic Council) or UKCP (UK Council for Psychotherapy).

For BPC, use http://www.psychoanalytic-council.org

For UKCP, use www.psychotherapy.org.uk

For CBT, you could find a chartered psychologist through the BPS (British Psychological Society) www.bps.org.uk, or a practitioner through BABCP (British Association for Behavioural and Cognitive Psychotherapies) http://www.babcp.com

Summary

If you are struggling with your emotions and the impact of the disease on your quality of life, your relationships and your mood – you are not alone. There is expertise out there, there are others who have struggled with these issues before and have been helped. Ask for help early rather than struggling on your own.

Crohn's disease from the patients

The following stories are accounts from individuals who have experienced anxiety and/or depression as a result of their Crohn's. They talk through their experience and the steps they took to help them feel better.

Deepan

Deepan is 23 and studied computer science at Kingston University. Here he describes a difficult time in his Crohn's story.

"Depression set in after my second attempt at Humira (Adalimumab) failed. I was on it happily for about 12 weeks. I then went in for my week 14 injection. I usually have my injection in halves – first half of the injection and then five minutes later, I take the second half. Luckily, I have an aversion to stabbing myself with needles, so I was at hospital in the physiology department, being stuck with the needle the first time. My IBD nurse specialist went back into the main area, and within 20 seconds, *anaphylaxiss* [1] set in. My throat was closing up and my eyes were going hazy. Allergic reaction. Another medication in the "not compatible" pile.

At this point, I thought "why me?" I had been on about four different trials, and had most courses of medication available, and the medications have either worked for a while, and then stopped, or had no effect whatsoever.

> **1. Phil (Surgeon) says:**
> Anaphylaxis is a severe allergic reaction. It can be very serious but medications to treat anaphylaxis are always available when drugs like Adalimumab are given and the majority of reactions are far less severe.

I became a recluse, not going out, spent money on absolute rubbish, hung out with the wrong crowd and kept everything bottled up. During this time, I spent a lot of time either in my room, or in my car. When I get into my car, I feel free, I feel invincible, untouchable. Before I began studying childcare, I spent nearly 18 months being lazy at home, Sunday to Friday and working Saturdays. Daytime TV, the sofa and the microwave were my best friends.

I felt scared and alone; like no one understood what I was going through – and most of my friends and family didn't, so I had no one to turn to. The fear of my pain and condition kept me indoors and close to the bathroom and my painkillers. Friends' phone calls became few and far between as I realised that most people would only call if/when they needed things. The friends that I would talk to every few days started careers and became busy and unable to commit the same amount of time as they did before.

I even felt self-conscious of myself because of the effects of the medication. The steroids had stunted my growth, made my bones brittle, and being open to any and all infections from the azathioprine suppressing my immune system. I missed out on a few family holidays as well. Things did not look good at all.

Being at home and spending money became a habit, and debt became a problem. I began to hide it, and chose only to repay the minimum, just enough to get me to the next month.

Things began to snowball, until I was getting phone calls from the bank demanding payments; and when my parents found out, I was forced to go to work five days a week to pay for their bailout. This didn't even make me flinch, so I went out and I thought nothing of it. I enjoyed going to work, and had the impression I was getting paid to do something I enjoyed.

What hit home was that all my friends were moving on with their lives and careers, and I was being left behind.

Once I saw that my friends were moving on without me, I had to cement plans. I decided to go back into IT. I've enrolled myself onto an accreditation course and

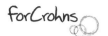

have built relationships with key people at work to help. Now that I have a goal to work towards, it's keeping me focused and freeing my mind somewhat of stress. I'm not as tired when I get home from work, and I'm more sociable outside of it. I would go out to the pub, meet friends for dinner and just generally enjoyed the company of other people again.

My work has improved. I've found myself becoming more productive with my time, building and maintaining new relationships within my studying life and also my working life. I'm the type of person who doesn't do well doing nothing. I'm not the type of person to wake up at noon and watch television until the early hours, and that's why I get out of the house seven days a week.

The one thing driving me is my course and the people I work with. They drive me, and constantly encourage me to be the best I can. I've met people within my company that I would never have met otherwise, and have really found the support I was so desperately searching for."

Claire

Claire is 23 and a nursing student. She is single and was diagnosed with Crohn's eight years ago.

"I was diagnosed with Crohn's at 15, but at about 18 or 19, the reality of Crohn's was hitting home. I guess you could say I was in denial from 15-18, and at this point, I acknowledged I had depression.

I have struggled with depression over time as it comes in waves, and I have only just started taking antidepressants after a mini breakdown – when I finally realised I couldn't cope any longer.

Crohn's is an embarrassing disease that can take a good deal of your social life away. My depression got worse at uni when I found I couldn't drink alcohol and was too tired to go out. I have had a constant battle with my family who don't understand why I'm depressed. They still *believe I was cured when I had my surgery* [2] and don't see any reason why I should be unhappy.

> **2. Phil (Surgeon) says:**
> This is a sad misunderstanding. As Claire implies, she was not cured – Crohn's is always with someone once diagnosed and recurring symptoms are common with further surgery sometimes required. Information produced by the charities mentioned in this book or via the doctors and IBD nurses can help not just the patient understand Crohn's disease, but family and friends too

I have found it hard to talk about depression with others as I feel there is so much stigma attached to it.

The only people who do understand are my fellow Crohnies on Twitter, as the majority of them also suffer with depression as a result of Crohn's.

I don't have much confidence in myself and often struggle to talk to new people. The main symptoms were *lack of self-esteem, tiredness, feelings of failure and not concentrating properly. I had no desire to do anything* [3].

Anti-depressants have definitely helped and I have also been seeing a counsellor since September, which has helped me learn things about myself and how to deal with Crohn's and the negative effects it has.

I still struggle on a daily basis as I'm constantly in fear of my disease coming back, which makes me worry – every time I feel pain, I'm afraid it's the disease coming back.

> **3. Phil (Gastro) says:**
> These are classic symptoms of depression and a discussion with the GP or gastroenterologist is worthwhile, as they can put you in touch with helpful services as Dr Stern has described above.

I also struggle with body image issues because of my scar and confidence, but I feel that if I continue to work with my counsellor over time, I can make big changes to improve my life.

Despite all this, I feel I am a stronger person since being diagnosed. I have learnt to be grateful for everything I have and live life to the full – although my disease restricts me in some ways, it does not define me! I have met so many inspirational people since my diagnosis, who have inspired me to campaign for IBD awareness worldwide. I actively help run a youth club for children with IBD. I also organise my own meetings for people with the disease – we get together and support each other. I don't know where I'd be without the support from my fellow Crohnies.

Crohn's disease has taught me so much, and has inspired me to train as an IBD nurse so I can continue to help others in the future."

Kelsea

Kelsea is 22 years old and a student midwife. She was diagnosed aged 20 and has undergone several operations for various aspects of her Crohn's disease.

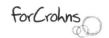

"When I was first diagnosed with Crohn's disease, I actually felt surprisingly OK about it. This was due to feeling grateful that I finally had a diagnosis after months of tests, as well as having a very close friend who was diagnosed a year before me who was coping well, so I thought: well, I'll be fine! Even knowing that my colon was in such a poor condition, that I had to go on a diet of *Modulen and water for eight weeks, followed by having a laparoscopic right hemi-colectomy* [4], I still felt very positive. I was looking forward to the operation, as in my mind, this meant that the pain would stop. My operation was a success, and over a year on, I rarely have stomach pain or have to rush for a bowel movement.

However, a month after my hemi-colectomy, I developed a perianal abscess, and since then I have had numerous operations for fistulas. After the first abscess, I spiralled into depression. I felt like my life had been taken from me, everything was unfair and I was never going to get better. After family and friends started to comment on a change in my behaviour, I decided to go to my GP who referred me for cognitive behavioural therapy. It was a specific group session for individuals with chronic/long-term health conditions. This helped me dramatically, especially being around people who were also depressed due to their health. We *helped each other through the process.* [5]

Once this course was finished, I had a personal counsellor who I had weekly phone consultations with. I now feel much better in myself; I still have days when I feel down, but as a general rule, I am happy. If anyone with Crohn's disease feels like they cannot cope, the best thing is to go and see your GP as soon as you begin to feel this way. The longer you leave it, the worse it gets. If you feel you cannot go to your GP, there are charity organisations that can give you advice and support. We aren't alone, and Crohn's is only a part of our lives, we cannot allow it to take over!"

4. Phil (Surgeon) says:
Modulen is a diet which can reduce inflammation and is discussed in the Diet chapter. Kelsea also underwent removal of the right half of her colon by the key-hole method which is discussed in detail in the Surgery chapter.

5. Phil (Gastro):
it is often helpful to meet other people with the same condition to share experiences, advice and tips to help you 'get through' the worse times and maximise the 'best times'. If you would like to meet other people you can ask your gastroenterologist or IBD nurse if they know of any local support groups that can help.

Summary:

The stories in this chapter show the different ways that those with Crohn's have been affected psychologically and how they have felt able to seek help; whether through friends and social media support groups or through different forms of therapy. They all discuss the importance of seeking help and acknowledging that you don't need to tackle the condition alone.

Tips and suggestions

- **If you feel your Crohn's is getting you down, try to speak to someone you feel comfortable with**
  This might be a family member, friend, GP, IBD Nurse or gastroenterologist.

- **Consider whether social media might be something to explore.**
  It can offer a community of 'Crohnies' with whom you may find it easier to share aspects of your life but beware that many people use the opportunity to discuss their most difficult times and it can be quite distressing seeing all those accumulated on one Facebook page. Use social media with caution but if you are interested, search for Crohn's chat forums, groups on Facebook, or use #Crohns on Twitter to find an online community that suits you.

- **Your GP may recommend counselling, medication or 'talking therapies' like cognitive behavioural therapy (CBT) or psychoanalytic therapy.**
  Discuss the different options in detail to find out what feels right for you.

- **Remember that many others with Crohn's have also battled with anxiety and depression and sought help to get through it**
  You are not alone in this.

Section 3

Crohn's disease from the loved ones

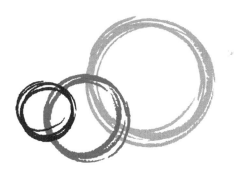

189

Parents

The following accounts all come from a range of parents whose children have Crohn's disease. The parents all describe a mixture of feelings from powerlessness and anxiety to relief at a diagnosis and pride at how well their children are coping. All of them find their own ways of supporting their children and hope that by sharing their stories, it might help you as parents too.

Helen

Helen is 57, married with two kids and is retired after enjoying a career as a science technician. Her daughter was diagnosed with Crohn's when she was 14 and has undergone four operations.

"Right then, where do I begin? The saga that was finally given the name of Crohn's first reared its ugly head, we believe, when our daughter Cassie was eight years old and started complaining of abdominal pain that was attributed to stress by two GPs and then irritable bowel by a third.

We muddled through for five years, but then when she was 13, she began to tell us that she could not eat and felt sick much of the time. I have to confess that as we had only recently succeeded in overcoming Anorexia Nervosa with our elder daughter we, along with our GP, initially assumed that Cassie was adopting some kind of shadow condition as the worry about her sister had hit her hard.

As she continued to lose weight over several months and was now 14 and complaining of severe pain and missing a lot of school, we started to realise that there was more to it and when she spent Christmas Day curled up in pain and unable to eat at all, we resolved that we had to act. The following day, we called in a doctor who after initially suspecting a kidney infection, eventually arranged for hospital admission for *suspected appendicitis* [1].

When Cassie was taken to theatre, she was frail and underweight – a shadow of the girl she had been before this escalation of symptoms. She was away in surgery longer than we had been led to expect, but I was told not to worry as all was going OK. When she was ready to return to the ward, I was collected by a nurse and the surgeon (Cassie's was the only operation, as it was Christmas), who told me that they had not found appendicitis but had I heard of Crohn's disease? This was one of those things that one hears of but doesn't really register until it gets closer to home.

I was reeling – she had about one metre of small bowel removed and there was more diseased bowel that the docs fully expected would continue to give her trouble.

I cannot sufficiently convey what it was like to sit all night watching Cassie (dad was at home with our other daughter). She was absolutely white, though she is naturally a very pale redhead, had a *naso-gastric tube* [2], was on strong intravenous antibiotics and was drifting in and out of a very hazy consciousness, wanting to know why she was hooked up to tubes that she had not expected, and trying to pull out the ng tube. I was so very fortunate that a member of the night nursing staff found me a small booklet issued by the National Association for Crohn's and Colitis (now CCUK), which armed me with a little knowledge so I was able to answer her questions as soon as she was ready for them.

10 days later, we went home, but Cassie was still very weak and needed me to sleep in her room as she was scared of being alone because she needed so

> **1. Phil (Surgeon) says:**
> An acute attack of Crohn's, especially when it affects the end of the small bowel (terminal ileum), can appear a lot like acute appendicitis until surgery is performed and the diagnosis is made.

> **2. Phil (Surgeon) says:**
> A tube passed through the nostril into the stomach which drains the stomach and the bowel like a siphon. It is used when the bowel is lazy (called ileus) or blocked, to relieve back pressure and avoid vomiting. They are very useful and generally make patients feel a lot better but can be uncomfortable to put in.

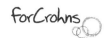

much help. As she recovered, she was on steroids, azathioprine and a low residue diet and gained more weight than she was happy about, but this did all keep her going. Slowly her strength returned and she was able to return to school, but there was more to come. Later that year, she suffered an obstruction due to inflammation and was back in hospital for a week, and at 18 had more surgery, this time to perform a stricturoplasty, remove adhesions and *redo her hemicolectomy* [3].

> **3. Phil (Surgeon) says:**
> This is a common set of procedures for people with Crohn's where the small bowel becomes narrowed and new inflammation often occurs at the site of a join made at the previous operation. See the Surgery chapter for more detail.

She missed a lot of school over these years, but was able to sit both GCSEs and A Levels and attained great results. Her social life had been severely curtailed as she suffered such bad fatigue that she was often asleep by seven in the evening, but she managed to join a drama group and was even on stage the day before her admission for obstruction.

Following all of this, Cassie then had 10 years in remission that allowed her to go to uni and have a near-normal life. She still had fatigue issues and episodes of nausea and pain, but on the whole she had a good time, including getting married and buying their own home. Unfortunately the Crohn's flared up again when she became pregnant, and we had to watch her deteriorate over the next three years, as she would not allow herself to give in – denial having always been her way of coping with the reality of being sick.

Various drug regimens were tried but she failed to respond to them and finally, after having two more hospital admissions and investigations that revealed a severely inflamed colon, the decision was made that a permanent colostomy was the best option. Actually, by the time Cassie was admitted for the op, she was already obstructing, having continued to insist that she could soldier on. None of us could make her give in sooner and her resilience worked against her to some extent, as to me the doctors did not seem to realise how much pain she was suffering.

The outcome of the surgery was different to our expectations, as once in theatre it was found that the damage was a little higher than expected, so it was possible to retain Cassie's rectum and perform a loop ileostomy instead, meaning that she has an option for reversal in the future. Cassie was very distressed at first, when the result she had prepared herself for was changed, but then she developed an infection due to leakage from the remaining debris that hadn't been able to be cleaned out. She was very poorly and for a while wished she hadn't had the surgery, though we soon discovered that because she was obstructing anyway, she would have ended up in surgery even if it hadn't been planned. Once we understood all the technicalities of the surgery, we were able to see why things changed the way they did.

Cassie is doing really well now; her husband and little boy both accept the stoma as a part of life and they are all enjoying life together again. She is able to eat foods that she hasn't been able to consider for years and is having fun trying out 'new' foods. I don't know whether she will opt for a reversal – that will very much be her decision, but it won't happen soon. She is enjoying her renewed health too much and being a 'proper mum' (her words) again as she is able to look after the little one without help now. She is back at work full-time in her nursing post, though I still worry that it is too much.

It is hard to describe how it feels to be the parent of a child with *a chronic, incurable disorder* [4]. As a mother, the natural instinct is to make everything right and it feels like letting the child down when there is nothing that can make it go away. It is vital to get past this feeling in order to be able to give what help you can. Hugs go a long way and it helps to have an unending supply, as these are still welcome once that child reaches adulthood and continues to battle the disease along with trying to have a normal life and all that brings with it.

Over the years since my daughter was diagnosed, after emergency surgery at fourteen have become a stronger person. I have learnt much about Crohn's disease and have been able to help others when they have had to deal with the news that a family member has been newly diagnosed. I have gained enough knowledge to be able to pressure my daughter to seek help when she wasn't acknowledging that there was anything wrong, because her greatest way of coping is denial that the Crohn's exists in her.

> **4. Phil (Gastro):**
> Parents often feel a sense of guilt when their child is diagnosed with a chronic illness. Was it something they did – their genetics? The food they fed them? Of course, they should feel no guilt as it is not anyone's 'fault'. But the role a parent plays in helping to control their child's Crohn's disease in childhood through to being a young adult should not be overlooked. 'Transition clinics' help prepare both the parents and the child for managing their own disease in the future

Over the 16 years since her diagnosis, I have experienced more emotions than I would have thought possible. There has been worry and fear, frustrations, anger and more. The love that I have for my daughter has carried me through all of it, and despite being disabled through chronic illness myself, I have found strength and endurance enough to care for my daughter and grandson whenever necessary – during the four-year flare-up because it is impossible for her husband

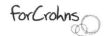

to work, travel for hospital appointments and ward visits and look after her little boy as well.

We will now hopefully all have a period of 'normal' life as Cassie now has a temporary ileostomy. Although this is one of the last resorts, it has given her back a freedom that she hasn't had for many years – much less running for toilets, no pain and eating almost anything she wants. It is wonderful to see her back to good health and I understand her reticence about having a reversal anytime soon, so the most recent emotion is joy and happiness – and long may it last!"

Imelda

Imelda is 52, married with two kids and works as a lawyer. Her daughter was diagnosed with Crohn's when she was 18, and Imelda would describe it as 'moderate' in severity.

"The elephant in the room"

"Clare, our daughter, had never had a day's illness in her life. She'd avoided all the childhood illnesses despite my best endeavours to expose her to the various viruses, hoping she'd get them and deal with them early in life, and be fit for school! She even managed to avoid them when her brother contracted them. She was strong, athletic and an Irish dancer who competed at World Championship level.

Shortly after her 18th birthday, and after returning from a school expedition to Africa, where she helped build a classroom (yes this was a fit young girl), my dad, her beloved granddad Tom died. I didn't then, but I wonder now, was this the trigger, the shock, the stress that kick-started the Crohn's intrusion into Clare's life and into ours?

This was also at the time she got her A Level results and moved to university in London.

During her first term at university, Clare became ill. She constantly suffered colds, sore throats and infections. We thought perhaps it was a case of her living the student life and burning the candle at both ends, but by Christmas 2009, we were becoming increasingly concerned.

Clare started to lose weight and the throat infections were getting worse. She was now missing a lot of time from university due to illness. We brought her home to get her well. Our GP said hers was the worst case of tonsillitis he had ever seen. Her tonsils were ulcerated. She was admitted to hospital and placed on IV antibiotics and things started to improve. Our GP was kind enough to follow up and ask how Clare was doing. We reported that she was going back to university. He said he was a little worried and suspected that there might be more to this tonsillitis. He suspected IBD. It was the first time I had ever heard the term, as he explained this was different to IBS. He wanted her to undergo tests, so he contacted the GP at the university and said Clare should be referred to a gastroenterologist.

> **5. Phil (surgeon) says:**
> Florid, frequent and multiple ulcers may be a sign of inflammatory bowel disease although mouth ulcers also appear in many people without Crohn's disease.

Within two weeks of her return, she was ill again. She quickly became confined to her room, too weak to walk without aid. Her *mouth was full of ulcers* [5] and she couldn't eat. She complained of incredible pain. I knew I had to get to her quickly and bring her home again.

When I saw Clare, I was shocked. The deterioration had been rapid. I took her to the GP on campus who immediately said she had to be admitted to hospital. I wanted her back at home and the GP agreed to phone our local hospital to tell them I was on my way, and to expect an emergency admission.

It all then happened so quickly. Clare was admitted to A&E, and the nurses, doctors, registrars and consultants all came rushing, keeping an eye on her, stabilising her, and treating her. There was no question my baby girl was sick.

Days of IV antibiotics, steroids, drugs, needles, poking and prodding followed.

Finally, on 4 March 2010, she was told she had Crohn's disease. *She shocked us by telling the consultant that she suspected she had this* [6]. While her condition had been deteriorating, she had researched every symptom she suffered and had concluded as much herself.

> **6. Phil (Gastro):**
> We often hear parents of young patients with Crohn's disease tell us that they have made multiple visits to the GP before a referral is made to the gastroenterologist. Although things are improving in recognition of the condition, persistence is key and often parents 'know' that something is wrong with their child that is being missed.

I had never heard of Crohn's disease. This was going to be a huge and steep learning curve. Even though we now had a diagnosis and we had been told it couldn't be cured, the fact that it would be a lifelong battle didn't register with me at the time.

I think perhaps I was too much in despair watching her pain and not being able to take it away. By now, I could count every bone in her body. You could see her rib cage, you could count her vertebrae. I took my 18-year-old daughter to the toilet, stroked her hair, rubbed her back… anything at all to try and ease her pain. I suddenly found myself again bathing her, my 18-year-old daughter, as I had done when she was a baby, too weak to take a bath and wash herself, too weak to wash her hair.

> **7. Phil (Gastro):**
> Every parent is different and accepting the illness can often be as hard for the parent as it can be for the patient. Education and support is key and the gastroenterology team alongside charities can support parents to overcome their fears.

Still I managed to maintain a brave face, though my heart was breaking. I had to be strong for her and for my husband and son who couldn't quite deal with it all. I only cried once when alone, and what reduced me to tears was the memory of hearing my 18-year-old daughter say: "I'm so sorry to put you through this, mum!"

The effect it had on the family was strange. I had to know and learn everything I could about Crohn's disease. I searched the internet, bought and read books, joined a national charity, became a volunteer for that charity and joined social network groups and sites to "meet" other Crohn's patients and parents. I started a small Crohn's charity myself, simply to raise awareness.

My husband is completely the opposite. He cannot accept that his "little girl" has an illness that can't be cured, that will cause her problems, flares, possibly surgery and a lifelong prescription to medication. He cannot talk about it. He won't talk about it. If she catches a cold, he worries and becomes very angry and *fearful that a cold is the start of something more sinister* [7].

My son became quiet around her and repeatedly asked me "is she going to die?"

Clare herself was comforted by me doing as much as I could to learn about Crohn's, though she never wanted me to tell her too much about it. I would drip feed information as and when she asked for it. I suspect initially she experienced a little denial that this was with her for life and life had changed.

Clare and I now discuss her Crohn's, and she is open and honest with me. She keeps it from her dad as she knows he can't cope and asks me to keep it from him too. We have agreed to tell her dad things on a "need-to-know basis"!

When Clare visits home now, life is just as it was, although there is always an unwelcome guest that accompanies her. That guest is the elephant in the room.

We all know it's there but when we're all together, we don't acknowledge it. We try to treat her as we always did, but perhaps we secretly watch her every move a little too closely, looking for signs of a flare, anything that might go unnoticed.

> **8. Phil (surgeon) says:**
> This is great advice. An open dialogue between the patient and doctor with supporting information from relatives can be incredibly useful for identifying new problems and monitoring response to treatment.

Taking a leap forward... Clare was stabilised and enjoyed two years in remission. She even returned to university and despite the odds and against medical advice, she worked all the hours she could to recover the lost time. During her last term at university, she experienced her first flare. Increased medication and a return to steroids meant she could continue and finish her degree. She awaits her results but is predicted to gain a 2.1 in English literature and politics. She has just secured her first job, working at the university where she studied, and we are so very proud of her.

Life with Crohn's disease does go on. You cannot bubble wrap your children, much as you might wish to, but be prepared to be their eyes, ears and voice when they are first ill or diagnosed. Be prepared to be a loud voice when it comes to talking to the medical experts! *Do not be afraid to question things. Do make notes and keep a diary of dates.* [8] I now keep a note and record the date of every change in medication or dosage, of every new symptom Clare experiences so that if I need to be Clare's voice again when she is ill, I can be and I can give a well-informed factual account of matters to her consultant.

So there it is, a very brief and fleeting glimpse of my experience with Crohn's disease.

As a parent, I want to be able to take away my child's pain. I can't. I want to reassure her that things will always be fine. I can't. I want to tell her that she will never face surgery. I can't. I want to tell the world about Crohn's disease. I CAN!"

Pam

Pam is 52, divorced with two children and works as a medical secretary. Her daughter was diagnosed with Crohn's when she was 19, and Pam would describe it as 'moderate-severe'.

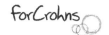

"My daughter Hannah has recently been diagnosed with Crohn's disease. She is 19 years of age and in her second year at university, studying event management.

She is my eldest child, I also have an 18-year-old son, Eliot, who is hoping to go to uni next year. Both of my children have sailed through their childhood years with only the usual minor ailments – coughs, colds etc.

Hannah completed her first year at uni with flying colours, she was happy, healthy and very pleased to have secured a house to live in for herself and four friends for their second year. It was at about this time that she began to suffer with diarrhoea, which we put down to food poisoning or a bug, but it continued and I suggested she register with a local GP. She was also getting quite bad stomach pains and was duly put on Codeine to control the pain, blood tests were taken which confirmed an inflamed bowel and a hospital appointment came through for December.

After suffering severe sickness one weekend a couple of weeks later, she rang me and I advised her to go back to her GP straightaway, who took more blood tests. She was now anaemic and had lost a stone in weight. I felt helpless that she was so far away, it's awful to have your daughter crying on the phone to you when normally she is bright and cheerful. Her GP advised her to attend A&E without delay. Hannah rang me and we took the decision for her to come home, and the next day we went to A&E at our local hospital, where I work as a medical secretary.

We saw three doctors that day, and eventually Hannah was admitted to the ward with a provisional diagnosis of Crohn's disease. It was almost a relief for Hannah to have confirmed what she already suspected, having read up on Crohn's on the internet, she was displaying the four main symptoms. I had also read up on the disease but somehow I couldn't get my head around the fact that my normally healthy daughter might actually have quite a debilitating condition.

Hannah was admitted at 1am, having been in A&E since just after 9am the day before. I was beside myself with tiredness, exhaustion and worry, but Hannah remained calm and cheerful throughout it all, knowing that finally she was in the right place and her treatment had started with a saline drip and steroids.

Myself, my husband and son spent most of that weekend at Hannah's bedside (in shifts) staying with her for as long as we could. She was having regular blood tests, intravenous drips, injections for pain relief etc. She was also taken off her beloved Codeine and the pain was almost unbearable, Paracetamol giving some relief. It's not nice to see your daughter suffering in such a way. The staff on the ward were all marvellous and the weekend passed in a blur of hospital visits, I didn't really have time to sit down and take in all the implications.

Although I did not get to speak to the doctors on the ward, Hannah was kept informed of progress. She was taken for a colonoscopy during the first morning on the ward, which confirmed Crohn's. As she is 19, she is classed as an adult, and so the staff spoke directly to Hannah rather than through us. At times it was difficult for me to hold back my emotion when I see my daughter in obvious pain. I was just glad I was there to hold her hand, stroke her hair, read to her and keep her spirits up.

I settled into a routine of popping in to see Hannah before work, at lunchtimes and then after work. I have been working at the hospital for almost a year, and I think Hannah felt comforted by the thought that I was just across the car park and it certainly made visiting so much easier. My nephew Matt is also a porter there, and he was brilliant about popping in to see Hannah whenever he could and making her laugh.

Each day she was improving. Finally after five days, Hannah was allowed to come home and Matt wheeled her out in a wheelchair. Armed with an array of literature and tablets, Hannah was just pleased to be home and started her daily concoction of medication. An MRI scan and second colonoscopy were booked, as well as a follow-up appointment.

We have all had to get used to Hannah being at home on a full-time basis and it has been quite a challenge to cook food that is nutritious but which doesn't give her a flare-up. Hannah has done a lot of research online, but I think it was most helpful when we met with the speciality nurse in the clinic, who basically went through everything with Hannah. Hannah's consultant also popped in to say hello and very kindly but firmly told her that she had to own the disease. They could give her the medication, but the more she did to help herself and keep a positive attitude, there was no

> **9. Lucy (IBD Nurse) says:** IBD nurses are a brilliant and invaluable source of information, support and advice for Crohn's sufferers, as well as being the fastest way to access specialist care when it is needed. Getting to know your local IBD nurse is one of the best pieces of advice.

reason why she should not resume a normal life and go back to uni in the New Year. *The IBD nurse also gave her a card with contact details, and she knows she can contact her at any time if she has a problem.* [9] Her medication has been changed and she is having weekly blood tests.

Hannah has started a blog, it's something she can channel her thoughts into and hopefully give advice and help to fellow sufferers. It seems to be creating a lot of interest and it is lovely to see Hannah with her old spark back.

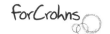

It's been a huge learning curve for us all, but I am so proud of the way Hannah has dealt with it all. Our lives will never be the same again, but if anyone was going to get Crohn's, then it may as well be Hannah as she has the strength and courage to deal with it in the best way possible.

It has been amazing the number of people I have spoken to who know of someone with Crohn's. It is far more common than we had realised. It is also genetic, though we have no knowledge of anyone in the immediate family who has suffered with it. There seems to be an awful lot of support for the person with the Crohn's but I, as a parent, have not been offered any support or advice. I am learning through Hannah how to manage it, but sometimes I feel quite inadequate as a mother. It's difficult to gauge how much I can do to help or whether I should let Hannah get on with it – after all, it's something she has got to learn to live with. I can only use my common sense and a mother's instinct, and hope that I get it right."

Diana

Diana is 59, married with one child and works as a family support worker. Diana's son was diagnosed with Crohn's when he was 14, and she would describe it as 'moderate' in severity.

"I took Will to hospital when he was about eight years old, with mystery stomach pains and fatigue – he had to lie down when he came home from school and often fell asleep. Will had gone down with glandular fever about three months previously and never seemed to regain his energy afterwards. It was a struggle to get the glandular fever diagnosed, our locum doctor at the time thought it was just flu and I had to press for a test. The consultant we saw for the stomach pains scoffed at my concerns that it was anything to do with glandular fever. She felt Will's stomach and pronounced that there was nothing wrong with him and that his mystery stomach pains must be emotional in origin. We were struggling at the time with Will's step-brother, who was beginning to show the first signs of schizophrenia, so we accepted this diagnosis. We were given family therapy, through which Will's dad's manic depression was also diagnosed.

Will's fatigue improved, but when he was about 14, he became very sick and could not stop vomiting. He was given medication for sickness by our GP, but did not improve despite further trips to the doctors over the next couple of weeks. His weight began to fall and Will's dad and I became very concerned. Eventually, I rang the doctor to say I was taking him to hospital and asked them to ring ahead and get a bed ready for him. When we arrived, Will could hardly walk as he was so thin and exhausted from retching continually. We were given a wheelchair for him and he was taken away for tests, holding a bowl to be sick in. Seeing him so thin, ill and frail as he was wheeled away, we really thought he had a terminal childhood cancer. It was one of the saddest experiences of my life, especially as I had nursed my mother through terminal cancer some years before.

We were lucky that the consultant Will saw also worked with one of the leading specialists in Crohn's. Will wanted to come home to await the results of tests, as he did not get the attention in hospital he was used to, with his frightened parents tending to his every whim. He could not stand bread or pasta and other wheat-based foods. We had to coax him with small amounts of his favourite foods – pomegranates was one of them and potato waffles! When Will's gastroenterologist gave us the diagnosis of Crohn's disease, his dad and I were so relieved. We could see Will was as well, although he had not expressed any fears about his illness. She stated that Crohn's was a very serious illness, and seemed perturbed that we were taking it so lightly – but we were all just so pleased that it was not a life-threatening condition, although these fears were unspoken. When I got home, I looked Crohn's disease up in the library and contacted a society that sent me all sorts of information, including gruesome pictures of sections of diseased intestines that had been removed. I kept this a secret from Will and my husband, and threw them away. I understood more about why the doctor was confused by our reaction, but I was resolved to stay positive and not think the worst.

Will was by now about four stone. He had been off school for a while and his friends understandably started to come round less and less. It was a very sad time seeing a young teenager so painfully thin and weak when they should be gaining confidence and enjoying their youth and strength. We were lucky that Will was referred to a specialist clinic in London. He was given an elemental diet to drink before meals. It was a bit like 'Complan' but it really seemed to work and settled his stomach, so that he could eat a little bit more at meal times. Steroids and later azathioprine helped. Although I was concerned about him taking these strong drugs, they were better than the alternative.

Will managed to get back on track with his education, and ended up with a 2.1 degree and a good job to boot. Not bad after all the disruption and time off school. He has stayed on the azathioprine for some time, still seeing his gastroenterologist as an adult. He has a close bond with the friends who knew

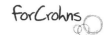

him when he was ill and has probably got up to things with them his mother would rather not know about. He came off all the drugs about three years ago, has never had any operations and has taken up physical fitness doing long-distance cycle rides for charity and regular cross training. We are immensely proud of all he has achieved and his positive and uncomplaining attitude throughout."

Siblings

The stories below describe what it's like having a sibling with Crohn's. The stories really differ, from those who live far away from their sibling and have to deal with the difficulties that distance brings, to those who know all too well what it's like having a sibling with Crohn's, because they have it too. They hope that their stories offer some support to you as a sibling and personal accounts that you can relate to.

Abigail

Abigail is 28, married and is a recently turned stay-at-home mum - having been a support worker. Her sister was diagnosed with Crohn's when she was 18 and has had two operations.

"There is ten years between myself and my older sister, but it's always felt like less. When I was young, she always felt like my friend despite the age gap. When Katie moved out, we still saw each other regularly and wrote long letters to each other. I was only eight when she was diagnosed, so my memories of the event are vague. Through conversations since, I know she had visited the doctor more than once before diagnosis and was either brushed off or given a variety of incorrect conclusions. When she was diagnosed, I remember her being rushed away in immense pain. An operation soon followed.

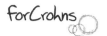
I'm sure I remember the years that followed the operation, my sister being active and happy. She worked, laughed and had fun. I think she was relieved that she had a name for her condition, so she could no longer be accused of being a malingerer, but she seemed to eat well and be able to carry on with every day activities like anyone else.

My sister is now 38, and those times seem like a lifetime away. I've lost track of the different procedures she has undergone and medications and diets she has tried. She hasn't been able to work for many years and has lost a huge amount of weight as a result of the condition. Crohn's and the drugs it has been treated with have created other issues such as kidney problems and arthritis.

For many years now, we have lived a couple of hours apart, so seeing each other has lessened to a few times a year, and contact through phone and text is sporadic. My sister has a very supportive husband who has been there since the very beginning of the condition, so I know she is in safe hands. This however does not prevent me from worrying regularly about her. Ties that bind sisters cannot be broken by distance. She has undergone operations since that she was warned could be fatal. I can recall clearly waiting by the phone, feeling sick to my stomach for it to be over and successful.

For many years, my sister and brother-in-law tried to get pregnant, which was made nearly impossible by her illness and the problems that went with it e.g. *polycystic ovaries.*[1] When I became pregnant with my first son, although I knew she would be happy for me, I couldn't deny the apprehension I had about telling my big sister how I had become pregnant with ease when they were struggling. Despite none of us believing it was ever possible, she did become pregnant and gave birth by caesarean to my perfect niece. I felt overwhelming happiness for her and hoped and wished to my core that she would go full-term and the baby would be healthy. She was of course monitored during pregnancy and medications were adjusted accordingly. When she was pregnant, my husband and I wanted to try for our second child but I insisted that we wait for my sister to give birth. After waiting for so long for this, there was no way I was going to steal her thunder, especially when we had no idea how her pregnancy was going to go. We began trying immediately after Freya was born.

My sister is so thin and gets tired very easily. This, along with everything else has meant that I worry about her, especially when I can't just pop in to see her. I

> **1. Phil (Surgeon) says:**
> Polycystic ovaries are not specifically related to Crohn's disease. The impact of Crohn's on fertility is discussed in the Having Children chapter.

worried even more when I imagined her at home with a baby while her husband had to work all day. I longed (and long) for her to move back closer, so I could pop round and help with chores or watch the baby while she rested or take her out in the car. I feel protective over her, but feel utterly helpless being far away and having my own responsibilities taking up my time, making it harder to visit. In spite of her illness pulling her down, she is doing a wonderful job of being a mother and Freya appears to be growing into a healthy, intelligent and happy little girl.

For those who know someone who has this horrid, incurable disease, it's easy to feel helpless. Part of me would like to be proactive, research the disease and different therapies, medications and remedies that may be appreciated by some. If this is relevant for you, definitely try. My sister however, is headstrong, and has lived with it for so long that she owns a book that lists thousands of medications, so whenever a doctor or specialist suggests anything, she looks it up. I think this probably gives her a bit of control over the disease, and prevents the professionals giving her something that she knows herself (because who knows her body better than her) will not work, is not relevant or has been tried before. Her file by now, you can imagine, is very large and some health professionals can miss what has been previously tried. So she doesn't need me looking up new therapies when she's heard and read it all before.

I took part in a sponsored Crohn's walk several years ago, which made me feel like I was doing *something* at least. Apart from that, all I can do is make sure she knows I'm thinking of her and I'm here and that I love her. It's simple but with this complex, incurable disease, all a sibling can do is keep their arms and their door open."

Ruth

Ruth is 57 and is divorced with two kids. She works as a bookkeeper. Her sister has had Crohn's for over 30 years, and has had a number of operations.

"My sister was diagnosed with Crohn's when she was 19 and I was 15. Nobody in our family had heard of this disease. I didn't really understand what was happening or what having Crohn's meant. I was so worried as I could see her

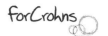

getting worse and there was nothing I could do. However, after major surgery, life returned to relative normalcy.

There were ups and downs, but on the whole she was not too bad.

When I was diagnosed at the age of 25, I knew she would be a great support, knowing what I was going through. She was devastated though, knowing what I was going to face.

The good thing was that we could discuss our symptoms and go to check-ups together. We had a disease in common and although it was a horrible thing, at least we had each other.

The hardest time came very recently. In November 2012, she had a major flare-up. After several tests, it was decided she needed surgery. This was a major blow and the surgery took its toll on the whole family. She was in intensive care for three days and the surgeon said the op had aged him! What about us?! It was definitely the worst time of my life. I was so frightened and worried for her. She was in hospital for nine weeks and I was there every day, trying to ensure I asked the professionals all the questions I had.

High temperatures followed with infection after infection. She lost three stone in weight. There was *a huge, deep abscess which had to be drained surgically* [2]. So again, another big op. obviously this was terrible for her, but as her sibling, it felt just as bad. I was so worried during this time, I really don't know where I got my strength from – although my children and her close friends were a tremendous support.

A drain was fitted which had to have a stoma bag covering it. While in intensive care, the stoma nurse asked me to look at it. How I didn't pass out is anyone's guess! But it was decided that when she left hospital – as she usually lives by herself – she would come and stay with me. Neither of us realised that this would end up being for over three months, or that I would be changing the stoma bag every day or two.

2. Phil (Surgeon) says:
This is one of the risks of surgery – patients with Crohn's tend to have a higher risk of complications after surgery including infections and delayed healing. We try to drain abscesses like this without resorting to another operation or simply treat them with antibiotics but sometimes there is no alternative to another operation.

Not only was it dreadful seeing her so weak and thin, but I was drained from the pressure of looking after her. Although, I admit, each time I changed the bag, I felt proud that I had done a good job when there was no leakage. What was also difficult was that I was trying to be strong for her, and not look worried every time there was another complication, trying to provide reassurance at each twist and turn.

Unfortunately, *she then developed a hernia* [3] so large she looked pregnant, so yet again another op and then back to me! Obviously I love my sister dearly, but by now, I was getting fed up with this whole cycle of changing her dressings and worrying about whether there would be light at the end of the tunnel – it was beginning to take its toll on me. Obviously stress is a trigger for Crohn's and I was also utterly exhausted. I came out in severe eczema and psoriasis, and needed steroid treatment myself.

> **3. Phil (Surgeon) says:**
> Another risk of surgery, when bulging occurs at the site of a scar from a previous operation. Surgery is the only way to deal with a hernia although they can also often be left alone with little risk or impact on a patient's life.

Also, at the back of my mind was – what if I needed another surgery? Would I have the same complications? Numerous surgeries? Infections? Not nice thoughts.

Well, I am glad to report that only this week – 10 months after the first op – there was no leakage from any of her wounds. Yipeeeee! Maybe life would get back to normal after all. There is no let up as you have to live with on-going symptoms, but we have each other for support and know the other understands what we go through – as only sufferers can."

Holly

Holly is 28 and works as a policy and communications manager. Her sister has had Crohn's for six years and she would describe it as 'moderate' in severity.

"My younger sister was diagnosed with Crohn's disease. I didn't have a clue what it was. I'd never heard of it before, but it sounded bad. It looked bad. It had put her in hospital for a few months. I needed to know more.

Speaking to close family members, nobody knew what it was, nobody had heard of it. I didn't get a chance to speak with the doctors, and none of my friends knew about it. After visiting my sister every day in hospital, caring for her and seeing what it was doing to her, I needed to find out more. So I decided to do my own research. Maybe looking back, searching the internet wasn't the best place to start. It brought up a lot of information, some of it very scary and not what I wanted to hear. Nevertheless, I wanted to be armed with all of the facts, rather than bury my head in the sand. So I did my research, and tried to help her through it.

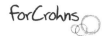

At first, she didn't want to discuss it. She still doesn't really. It was very hard to raise the subject with her; she made it clear that it was not up for discussion. I found it difficult not to be able to talk like we used to. So I decided to use humour. Making her laugh about the scary things that were happening to her really worked. We would joke about how she'd become such a "fussy eater" and how often she went to the toilet. We'd giggle about her "poo diary" and laugh about the amount of pills she was taking. I'd sit in hospital with her for hours and chat about what else was going on in the world, what friends were up to, what fun things we were going to do when she got better.

It is now very normal to see my sister avoid certain foods and to take medication daily. It is very normal for us not to discuss Crohn's anymore. If she wants to talk about it, she will. She knows I love her and I'm always there to talk if she ever wants to. She is still my little sister, that hasn't changed.

The experience with my sister has led me to be acutely aware of Crohn's and colitis. When I first met my partner (now friend), I picked up on the signs almost immediately. I didn't mention it initially; I didn't want to make either of us feel uneasy. But when the subject was raised and I spoke about my sister, I think we both felt relieved. I understood a little of what he'd been through. I didn't need to question why he had eating habits that were different; I didn't need to ask why he ate so many bananas every day or took longer to finish each meal. I didn't need to make a big deal of the scars on his body from his operations. I think he was self-conscious about the scars at first. To be honest, I hardly even noticed them! Together we taught him to be proud of them; they were a physical mark of what he'd been through. They made him unique and I loved him even more because of them. I admired his courage and strength.

With him it was different. Once we'd got to know each other, he was OK talking about his experience. He was open to sharing his worries and concerns. That really helped me to understand what my sister had been through and just how hard it must have been for her. It helped me to understand that people deal with it in very diverse ways. He taught me that whatever way each person chooses to deal with it is the right way for them, and you have to respect that. It is important to have someone to talk to about it, but equally, to have someone there to give you a hug and change the subject.

It is good to have people who've got your back. I'm glad my sister knows that no matter what, we will always be there for her. Being there from diagnosis made it easier. It was a shared experience. Trust is vital, and that builds over time. I'm sad that I didn't know my now friend when he was diagnosed. That I couldn't prove to him that I'd always be there for him through illness, operations, colostomy bags, whatever life threw at him. I'd get very upset when he'd worry that I wouldn't be there for him if he got ill again. I really hope he came to realise that no matter what, I will always be there for him. I will always love him and I will never ever let him down.

Of course there are challenges. Daily challenges like how close is the nearest toilet, have you got enough medication on you, is there access to food that won't cause a flare-up? Then there are longer-term challenges. Even going on holiday is a challenge – what is the water quality like, will there be food that is edible, will the person you're traveling with look after you properly if you get ill?

Crohn's and colitis affects all aspects of life. It causes confusion and uncertainty. It affects work, home, family, and friends. But sometimes that isn't a bad thing. It makes you and the people around you tougher. It helps you find out who your true friends are. It makes you appreciate life more. Yes it changes relationships, but most of the time it makes relationships stronger. And together with love, support, and humour, you get through it. One day at a time."

Partners

The below stories describe the experience of having a partner with Crohn's and range from those who knew about the diagnosis before meeting their partner to sharing the whole experience of diagnosis. They reflect openly and honestly about some of the challenges and hard times as well as their strategies and tips on how they have supported their loved ones.

Laura

Laura is 27, her partner was diagnosed with Crohn's six months ago. Laura would describe her partner's Crohn's as 'severe'.

"Hello I'm Laura, and I'm Craig's partner in crime (and Crohn's)

If I had to think of one word to describe how a partner of someone with Crohn's feels, it would be 'helpless'. This is also a theme I have noticed in spouse support areas in IBD forums too.

Quick number one fact. YOU ARE NOT A BURDEN. Remember that.

The word is helpless not, angry, upset, hopeless or mad.

I'm not angry at all most of the time, and certainly not at my partner because of Crohn's – other stuff like correcting my grammar when I talk is fair game! If I am mad or upset, it is at the people who have 'abandoned' us, who think that an IBD has control over when to get sick, can't be bothered or that they are functional. But that's just me.

I'm not feeling hopeless. I will never give up hope that we can beat this.

I will never give up hope that the meds will work and that we will come out stronger, ready to get our lives back or adapt to a new plan. I think I just feel a little helpless. I hate it when he can't sleep, or is in constant pain. We've recently found out that sometimes the IV steroid treatment makes him grumpy and that there is nothing I can do.

If he'd broken a leg? Stick a cast on it, wait for it to heal. Bang. Done. But this, this is different, there is no magic gut cast (yet). It's hard seeing your partner (or a buddy) in such a sickly state and not thinks "I wish it were me". not that **we** would cope better, it's just so they wouldn't have to suffer.

We don't want to keep nagging about meds, the importance of hydration, LowFlex diets, food, testing your patience etc. but *we* don't want you to get worse or be in any more pain.

I'm not without hope. I just sometimes feel a little helpless.

Craig slowly got sick, he was in so much pain that he struggled to get out of bed. He was very ill, after GP consultations, consultants, tests upon tests, he was a medical marvel to rival even Dr House's expertise. Work was impossible; he worked up until 2009, but after six months' sick leave, they had to let him go. He couldn't even leave the house.

My employer has been great with this and let me have time to visit him/carer's leave when needed.

Eventually we had the diagnosis of IBS-D (Irritable Bowel Syndrome with diarrhoea), then two years later, diagnosis of mild Crohn's colitis as well as secondary arthritis and gout.

Everything seemed to race past us. He missed out on friends' and family's birthdays, socialising, seeing distant relatives was impossible. Even though I wasn't sick, we became an insular unit. We wrapped ourselves in cotton wool while I worked two jobs and got out/did things when I could.

Some people left us behind, maybe thinking we were making it up? I don't know. I'd like to ask one day, but I sometimes think they just wanted to get on with their lives and visiting didn't fit in with that.

I am so grateful to those who have stuck by us, come to see us in little chunks, encouraged Craig and understood when we've had to turn stuff down.

I am so so so proud of him and everything he has achieved so far. He has been through so much these past few weeks, let alone years, and he has come on leaps and bounds, both mentally and physically. We've even managed, at one point, to

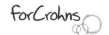

attend a wonderful wedding and an awesome reception, connect more with our friends, attend some family and friend events. Distance & wellness permitting

The hardest point was the hospitalisation and the lead up to it.

His symptoms started rapidly changing. Over three and a half months, he lost five stone, was in even more constant pain, then after a CT scan 10 weeks ago, the pain was so bad he had to sleep on an air-bed in the lounge. He could hardly move due to his arthritis and then started to have chest pains.

Two trips to A&E later, we found that the CT scan showed active IBD! I'd had to explain to an A&E consultant the difference between IBS and IBD and we got discharged with an IBD nurse number to call the gastro clinic. He got rushed in for an emergency colonoscopy and they found very active Crohn's. So much so, they admitted him into hospital.

Time altered terribly onwards. I constantly felt this need to be near him, I just wanted to get in his bed with him, cuddle him and tell him everything was fine. It changed him. The IV Prednisone changed him a lot. It made his needle phobia worse. He had the cannula in while he was out for the colonoscopy. His shape changed a lot. Very skinny but with the Pred moon face. Then the five blood transfusions, two plasma and time on IDA (intermediate dependency area) and the not knowing what was happening.

He got out on a Tuesday, the Saturday was our eight years together and the Sunday was the 10kforCrohn's charity event!

My key advice is to **persevere.** Persevere with your medical team. Persevere with fighting Crohn's. Either for yourself or your loved one. Cut yourself some slack as a partner, stuff is hard but it will get better. Don't let Crohn's cause resentment, don't smother; I tell Craig I have an open-door policy – you want to talk and have a hug? Awesome. Need 20 minutes on your own to get your noggin in gear? Cool. It's a hard balance between nagging and helping. Sometimes I do need to tell him to take his meds, not eat that etc. but I try not to harp on. Remember, it's not their fault they are sick, but don't let them walk over you or wallow for too long, everyone copes differently and has different symptoms that change daily.

IBD forums/websites, forCrohns and NACC really helped, getting a radar key and a 'can't wait' card is ESSENTIAL.

I have researched beyond belief! We brought Prof John Hunters book on IBD, which is good. Researched via medical books/journals/ejournals like pubmed, gone through Google relentlessly – however, a word of warning, you have to be aware of the sources.

Also, poop jokes are standard. Never be embarrassed about Crohn's and poo, because let's face it, everybody poops."

Juan

Juan has been married for two years, and his wife was diagnosed with Crohn's before he met her. Juan's wife has had several operations.

"I had never heard of Crohn's disease until I met my wife, Larissa. We met in Sao Paulo, Brazil, in May of 2011. I had been transferred by my company the year before, and she had come to teach English for six months. She was going to go back to the US in July, but we decided she would stay in Brazil, and in December 2011, we got married in Colombia. She had already told me about her condition, and I didn't really understand much about it, but as time went by and she explained it more, I got to understand it better. I didn't really think or feel anything about her having Crohn's at first. I read a little bit about it on the Internet, because I like to learn about these types of "little known" subjects and it helped me to understand the disease better. Because she always looked so healthy and full of life, I didn't consider it to be an issue. I was never worried that something bad might happen to her because of Crohn's. She explained she took medicine to keep it in remission and that made me feel more at ease.

When we got married, the insurance provided by my job also started covering her. I always go to all of her doctor's appointments and I translate everything in between her and her doctors, since I speak more Portuguese. This also helped me to understand Crohn's a lot better.

Her most recent flare-up since I've been with her happened in December 2012. She started experiencing a sharp pain near her anus. It happened while we were on a trip to Colombia to visit my family. We didn't think anything really bad about it and assumed it was a case of haemorrhoids. We bought a cream and it helped, but the pain never completely went away. After a few weeks, she developed a lump where the pain had started. The pain got so severe we had to go visit a doctor. He sent her a blood exam, but also didn't think it was anything bad. I have a friend who is a paediatrician and we sent him the results because we couldn't get a hold of the first doctor. My friend believed it was something more severe, maybe a flare-up, but he wasn't able to pin-point the real problem. We started searching on the Internet about the possible problem, and discovered it was an anal abscess. After that, we decided to go to the hospital.

I was really worried and afraid about the possible complications the abscess could cause, but I kept it all to myself and I didn't want to show her that I was

214

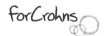

worried. She tends to stress a lot with her health and me also stressing out wasn't going to help. I'm able to keep my cool even in the most complicated situations, and I was always there to try to make her feel better and get her mind off our troubles. I did talk to some family members about it, because I know I can always count on them, but I decided to handle this situation by myself as much as I could. I don't think that reaching out is bad, I think it just depends on the type of person you are. I am very independent and I like to deal with my problems by myself, but I am also not afraid or ashamed to ask for help when I think I really need a hand.

I want to tell you a short story that will help me explain why I think and act this way. When my godfather was two years old, he got infected with Polio in both his legs. He is one of the most incredibly amazing people I know. He never let his condition affect him in any way in his daily life. He can drive a car, ride a bike, swim, dance, and when he was a kid he could even climb coconut trees using only the strength in his arms. He also has the greatest sense of humour. He could have grown up to be a completely different person, but he chose not to let his condition affect him mentally and spiritually. I learned from him that life is not always what you expect or want it to be, but that doesn't mean it has to be sad or depressing. There are so many things to appreciate and be thankful for. I carry that with me every single day of my life.

In the hospital, they confirmed she did have an abscess and she would have to undergo emergency surgery to drain the abscess and prevent it from bursting inside her body. We had a lot of trouble green-lighting the procedure with my insurance company (because we were out of the country) but in the end, she had the surgery. She was in a lot of pain and experienced a lot of discomfort during the weeks after the surgery. I was by her side every step of the way. It surprised me to know that this was only the beginning of the healing process and not the definitive solution, but as always, I kept up my good spirits and tried my best to not let her feel depressed by this.

The abscess had to be left open to drain for several months. Although, since the first surgery and until now, my wife has had to wear pads to catch the drainage, and it's very uncomfortable for her. When we got back to Brazil, we went to see her doctor. He said the surgery performed in Colombia had gone well and now we needed to wait for the abscess to continue to drain more. The doctor explained she would need to have two fistulectomy surgeries because her abscess had turned into *a fistula* [1] He also explained there was a possibility of her suffering from faecal incontinence after the procedures. I think this was the moment when I got the most worried, but

1. Phil (Surgeon) says:
This is a reasonably complex area of surgery and is discussed in more detail in the Surgery chapter.

fortunately our doctor was one of the best in the country and he did the surgeries in such a way that faecal incontinence wouldn't be a problem.

She had her last surgery about a month ago and the fistula has been fixed. She still has drainage, but the doctor said this would be normal for at least a couple more months. He explained that because of her condition and the medicine she takes (Immuran), it's impossible to predict when the drainage will stop. We are thankful that the worst part is over and she has been able to go back to her normal life.

It really hurt me a lot to see her going through so much. I always tried to remain strong for her, but there were a couple of moments when the stress was too much and I broke down. She couldn't work for a while, our insurance took some time reimbursing the money from the surgery in Colombia (which was quite a sum), and she was very limited in her physical activities... it was a complicated and tough year for us, but we hung in there and now we are back on our feet.

I think the most important thing we have is our unconditional love for each other. I always knew that whatever problems we had, it could always be worse. I am fortunate to be a person who always tries to keep his spirits up, and I try to do that for my wife also. Crohn's is a disease that can affect whoever suffers it in many different ways and without any warning when a flare-up is about to occur. But I guess that's what life is all about, dealing with the unexpected. The only thing you can really do is keep your spirits up, maintain a positive attitude, and always look forward to a better tomorrow."

Gillian

Gillian is 48, engaged with one child and works as a director. Her partner was diagnosed with Crohn's 18 months ago, aged 45.

"My partner, Paul, was diagnosed with Crohn's around 18 months ago, after a brief but severe illness. Our journey has been up and down, but overall we consider ourselves very lucky that Paul received a quick diagnosis and that his condition, to date, has not been too life changing. Nevertheless, there have been lots of moments when we felt utter despair, relief and fear – a real rollercoaster of emotions!

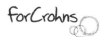

Paul is 46 and has been very healthy all his life. We first noticed Paul becoming ill during a holiday to Menorca. At first, we put it down to a 'Spanish tummy' style bug, but it persisted. Over the next few weeks, the symptoms became more severe and eventually Paul became very ill, unwilling to eat due to the effect it had on him and in lots of pain due to *fissures* [2] in particular. After self-diagnosing and self-medicating for a number of weeks, I eventually persuaded Paul to go to the GP. I recall that it was very frustrating watching him deteriorate so rapidly, yet be so reluctant to seek medical help. I think he had more or less convinced himself that it could be bowel cancer and was pretty terrified of what he might be told if he saw a doctor.

> **2. Phil (Surgeon) says:**
> Presumably anal fissures which make passing a motion extremely painful and are more common in people with Crohn's.

With hindsight, I feel that I could have done more to encourage and support him to seek help earlier. It was a very difficult time for the family. Paul was unable to work, was very ill to the extent that he needed a lot of care, and I had a demanding full-time job and a 10-year-old daughter to look after. Eventually, I had to ask my mum to come and stay and support Paul while I went to work.

After a couple of appointments at the GP, we were quickly referred to a consultant, and Paul received a diagnosis within days. Again, I consider us very lucky in that we *had private medical insurance* [3], so we got to diagnosis stage incredibly quickly. He was put onto steroids, which had an immediate beneficial effect. All we felt at the time was relief that it wasn't cancer and that we now knew what we were dealing with. After a couple of weeks, Paul started to regain some of the three stone in weight he had lost, and was able to slowly return to work on a phased basis.

> **3. Phil (Surgeon) says:**
> I think it's worth emphasizing that the main delay to diagnosis here was not the period from seeking help to getting a colonoscopy or appointment with a specialist and that even on the NHS Paul would hopefully have very quickly been diagnosed and had his treatment started.

Since then, it has been a learning experience. We immediately started to look for information and support. The Internet and social media sites have been superb sources for us both.

Our experience of the NHS system, that he has now had to revert to, is mixed. Lots of good people and good intentions but under severe pressure, poorly organised and not always there when you need them most. This has meant that other sources of support were even more vital to us.

We soon found lots of similar people – friends and acquaintances who had Crohn's and we either hadn't known about it or we did know, but didn't really understand it until now. They became invaluable sources of support too.

One of the issues for us both was that the symptoms of Crohn's are often embarrassing and not the normal dinner party-type conversation. It was difficult to explain to people how the illness manifests itself. I almost felt as if people would think that we were exaggerating the severity of the disease, as Paul was starting to look so 'well' again. This was a particular concern for Paul and his work. He used a great help sheet from the NACC site, which can be used to explain to employers what the effects of Crohn's can be.

The other biggest issues for us both since diagnosis have been:

Weight gain due to being on steroids for a year! Ironically making people think Paul was more healthy than was actually the case.

Fatigue – Paul has nowhere near as much energy and stamina now, which I have to be aware of and adjust to. Late nights are a thing of the past as sleep is a necessity.

Aching limbs – we think that his long-term medication causes this. I just have to put up with the moaning on this one!

Bloating and wind – this makes Paul feel very uncomfortable, especially if we are out for dinner at friends' houses, so again, I have to be conscious of this and know when we need to make excuses and leave.

Diet – I need to plan meals and try not to include too many of the ingredients that cause him bloating etc. when it's my turn to cook.

The smells (sorry, I couldn't resist this one!) – Paul has been banned from using the en-suite bathroom! We keep the bathroom window open for good ventilation!

Possible deterioration – I suspect that anyone diagnosed with an acute or chronic illness tends to think about the worst-case scenario. It can be quite mentally exhausting for me, trying to convince Paul that his diagnosis doesn't necessarily mean that he will go on to have part of his bowel removed or contract bowel cancer etc.

On the bright side, Paul is working full-time, exercising again, staying healthy and leading a pretty normal lifestyle. We are lucky to have had such good medical care initially, and such great support since."

Children

The stories below are from a number of people whose parents have Crohn's disease. They all have different experiences of the condition – for some, this includes sad memories or disrupted childhoods and for others, there may be particular aspects of their parent's condition that they found challenging. All of them are also able to reflect on the respect and admiration they have for their parent and the strength and courage they have witnessed.

Tasha and Josh

Tasha is 28 and works as a social worker and Josh is 25 and works as a talent manager. Their mother has had Crohn's for over 30 years. Here they tell their stories about the different ways it has affected them.

Tasha: "Crohn's disease is not particularly well known, and it is somewhat an embarrassing disease (to talk about as well as have). These two factors combined are where some of the main problems lie for both sufferer and family members.

My brother Josh finds that my mum's Crohn's affects him in one way in particular, which he constantly feels guilty about."

Josh: "A key example of my behaviour in regards to my mum's Crohn's disease, and the one that I will focus on, revolves around journeys. I outright refuse to travel long distance with her. For a recent family holiday abroad, I made sure I went two days after my mum and sister, so that I wouldn't travel with them. While away, I caught the bus after them and tried as hard as possible not to go anywhere where I'm not 100 per cent certain there was a toilet nearby (this is the case in London, too). If there are times when it is impossible for me not to travel with my mum, I spend the whole time sweating with worry.

The reason for this concern stems from experiences years ago. Sitting in a car, with your mum in the front seat, crying her eyes out, desperately needing the toilet and knowing she may not be able to find a place to stop, or that the traffic may not move, or somebody may not let her use their toilet, is heart-breaking. I remember watching from the backseat of the car while my mum was banging hopelessly on the front door of a friend's house, praying that she was in (she isn't), so that she could use the toilet, before running into a building site and having to plead with the builders to use one on site. These memories are some of the most painful and humiliating of my childhood. It is something that I decided I would never let myself be a part of again (once I got to the age where I could drive and travel separately)."

Tasha: "I think anyone who has to see someone they love go through both physical pain and the emotional aspect of embarrassment will understand some of these feelings, the heartbreak and powerlessness and sometimes the desire to remove yourself from the situation.

However, having a mum with Crohn's has also taught us many things.

For one, it has shown us strength of character, for we are constantly amazed by how much our mum goes through and puts up with, with so little fuss, ensuring it affects her as little as possible. I can't think of a better role model for us, both growing up and now.

Also I think it's taught both of us a real degree of empathy. I'd say we're both caring individuals and I personally have just changed my career to move into a "caring profession". I don't think I'd ever say that decision came directly from having a mum with Crohn's, but I do think many of the skills and values needed may have come from there.

Despite or perhaps because of my mum's Crohn's, we both have an incredibly close relationship with her and if anything, can see it as character building. It has certainly made me want to fight for the cause after being frustrated when so few people have heard of it.

In all, I think living with a relative with an illness of any kind will always be difficult at times, and perhaps affect certain parts of your life more than others,

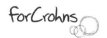

but for us I think it's brought us closer as a family and has given us someone we constantly admire."

Sarah

Sarah is 29, single and works as a writer. Her mother was diagnosed with Crohn's when she was 17 and has had a number of operations.

"Growing up with a mother with Crohn's disease wasn't very different from any other childhood I should imagine, except for small things that I hardly noticed. Mum rarely joined in things like sports days or being a class/school-trip assistant like other mums did. We didn't travel far from home very often. Trips to town were rare, so they were always big deals and we appreciated it more. We didn't have holidays, but that was maybe also due to us not being that well off financially, as mum couldn't work anymore, and had given up her job as a retail supervisor.

Yet she was always smiling, and never showed us she was ever in pain, but she would get very tired. She had been diagnosed at 17, in the 70s, back when it was unheard of, so no one really understood what Crohn's really meant. I, especially as a child, had no idea.

As I got older I began to notice more, and that's when I started to realise mum was different. That she had an "illness". She would be in horrible pain some days, and on one bad night, I remember her crawling up the stairs as she couldn't stand. It scared me, and made me realise that maybe she wouldn't always be around – not something a child should have to think about in primary school.

When I was 11, her condition drastically deteriorated, she was plagued with fistulas and abscesses, having to go into hospital to have them lanced and suffered from a lot of infections and complications. That year, she also went into hospital for her first ileostomy. She was so ill that we were told she may not even reach her 40th birthday. When she came out of hospital for the day for a small impromptu birthday party, it was the first time I saw a man cry – my grandfather saw her, and was in tears. She was so thin and gaunt, I was terrified.

She made a recovery, against all odds, and was back on her feet within months. She was never well from that point, and the ileostomy has resulted in a colostomy. My father had to carry on working as we had a mortgage to pay, so I helped her change and clean her stoma. As her health once again deteriorated, dad had to leave his job on a building site and become her full-time carer. We lost our house and moved to the nearby village to a council house. I was 13 and had never moved before, but I understood that there was nothing either parent could have done to change the situation. My elder sister took it a lot worse, and at age 18, she moved out.

Mum's condition stabilised for a few years, I continued to help dad to take care of her as I completed school. I went on to college and she became poorly again. There were complications with the stoma, and mum's own nutrition/ inflammatory levels. She had more operations resulting in *the colostomy being irreversible*.[1]

The doctors offered her a course of infliximab, back when it was a new drug, and she happily agreed, always willing to try new things to live a healthier life.

Life seemed to improve a lot, mum was much healthier and it was the most well I had seen her

> **1. Phil (Surgeon) says:**
> We often make stomas in order to protect a join in the bowel that we have made and such stomas are reversible when the join has healed. Sometimes stomas are made because the bowel beyond has been removed or sometimes further surgery is simply too dangerous to contemplate. In these situations a stoma may be permanent. Your surgeon will always discuss this with you before an operation if a stoma is likely. This is discussed in more detail in the Surgery chapter.

in years. She was making plans and starting to talk about trying things she hadn't done before due to being ill or being embarrassed by her stoma.

Then her specialist told her that during her last operation, a tumour had been found and that a biopsy had revealed she had cancer. A complication from the result of nearly 30 years of Crohn's damage to her tiny frail body. She had just months left. We were all devastated. The ghost of Crohn's had hung over us my whole life, but just when it seemed to have lifted, it crashed down. She died on 13 January 2002, aged 46. I was 18.

There isn't a day that goes by when I don't miss her, especially now that I'm also becoming sick and am facing the same demon. I wish she was here for advice on the bad days, but I learnt so much from her, about fighting Crohn's, and at least I have that.

It has definitely affected me in my relationships with others, I'm terrified of losing another member of my family. I had a lot of issues growing up, with going to school or staying at friends' houses. I was terrified something would happen while I was gone – that she would go into hospital or would die while I was away and I wouldn't know. I would have nightmares and cry myself to sleep. I had a

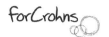

social worker for a small time. My truant levels were shocking, as all I wanted to do was stay home.

I had seen some horrible sights while caring for her, changing her dressings, cleaning her stoma and the one that always sticks in my memory is a later one when her colostomy was filled with blood, and when she used the commode to urinate, it was also filled with blood. No child should have to see their parent suffer like that.

But on the flip side, my mother is still the most inspirational person in my life. She was amazingly strong through everything she endured – the tests, the operations, the needles, the tubes – all done with a smile on her face and a joke made. She would always say that somewhere out there was someone suffering far more than she was. I have never met anyone who has equalled her kindness and positivity. If there was someone else on the ward with Crohn's, she was happy to sit with them and chat, or explain something the doctors hadn't. She had suffered at a time when Crohn's was still being understood, and she was one of the first supporters of awareness.

The whole experience has also helped me to appreciate the people around me, and my own life, because life is short and we should appreciate each day, as it is precious and not guaranteed.

My advice to other children of sufferers is to be patient with your parent. If they can't do what other parents can, please try to understand and not get angry or frustrated with them. Be sympathetic, and above all, supportive. If you can help them, even if it's something small such as walking the dog for them, then do it! Treat each day with them as a gift, as, trust me, *you will miss them so much when they are gone.*" [2]

> **2. Phil (Surgeon) says:**
> It is important to note that this situation is not common in Crohn's disease. Most people with Crohn's suffer from it but live with it and most readers are unlikely to face the desperate situation Sarah describes.

Emma

Emma is 25 and a full-time mum. Her mother has had Crohn's for over 25 years and has had a number of operations.

"My mum had an operation about four years ago, when I was 19. It scared the hell out of me because my mum was in hospital for nearly two months. She had originally gone to visit the GP with pain and they thought it was an appendix problem, but she found out it was her Crohn's. After she was in for two months, she came out but then had to go back in for a week because it got infected.

I had to do a lot of growing up because I didn't know what it was all about. I had all my family help while my mum was in hospital, plus the help of my sister who is three years younger than me. I was scared when my mum was in hospital because it meant I was the one who had to look after everything.

After my mum came out of hospital completely, I made sure she wasn't doing too much – and just made her feel like the queen! It still worries me today, as I don't know if it will come back the way it did or not. She is on medicine for life now, and is left with a scar on her belly, but is coping fine. I'm glad I still have my mum, I would not change her for anyone!"

Katie

Katie is 15 and at school. Her mum was diagnosed with Crohn's when she was eight years old and has had two operations.

"My mother has suffered with Crohn's disease for as long as I can remember. There was never a time where she was simply fine, it has just always been there. From a very young age, I have had to deal with the stress of a mother disappearing in and out of hospital quite frequently through no fault of her own. Within the past seven years, my mother has had two major surgeries and has been in and out of hospital a countless number of times. The effect of a having a loved one in hospital caused me to become very down and depressed, this was simply due to the fact that she was filling my thoughts, not that she doesn't anyway, but just more so when she's in hospital, causing me to overthink and worry about her. If it came to her going into hospital to stay for a period of time, I'd go about my normal every day school life, being a shadow of my former self, and then spend the evening with my mother at the hospital, which quickly became the highlight of my day.

My only positive thought from my mother having Crohn's disease is that this disease is not terminal. I'm still so lucky to have my mother, whereas some people I know don't, or are losing their mum. It makes me happy to know I still have her; every day I wake up knowing she's the same woman as the day before. It still frustrates me to watch my mum go through so much pain though, because there is no way I can

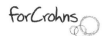

help her. When it comes to her illness I am helpless. With my mum being someone as strong as her, who doesn't let it affect her as much possible, I know she doesn't deserve it. It used to put a complete halt to family holidays/days out because my mother was simply too afraid to go out with the pain her Crohn's was giving her. This in turn slightly ruined it in my younger years as a child. But now I am older, and more understandable to such things like my mum's disease, I understand that my mum and dad have still managed to give me and my sister the best (and I mean the best) life possible, despite the setbacks we and my mum have had to go through.

Don't get me wrong, me, my mum, sister, and dad have had some absolutely amazing days through spending time at the hospital. Sounds weird, right? But it's true. I'll always remember the good days spending time with my mum, sitting on the edge of her hospital bed playing with the controls that moved the bed, up, down, head up, head down, end up, end down – oh how annoyed my mum would get with me and my sister. We couldn't help it though, we were young! We would always sneak food in for my mum, because my mum being who she is, absolutely hated hospital food – I mean who doesn't?!

Sometimes things got really serious and bad due to the Crohn's flaring up, causing her to have major surgery. Her latest surgery in January 2012 was especially hard because at first, they told us she would have to stay in over Christmas, which of course my mum was reluctant to do. She wanted to be at home with her family over Christmas, even if it meant being in pain. There was so much stress, to see if she was OK, helping her all the time especially after her surgery; I felt like a nurse helping my mum, which I was glad to do as it became the highlight of my day seeing her. Having a mum in hospital put so much stress on my dad, though it is easier now in our teenage years, because my sister and I can more or less fend for ourselves. Though it didn't stop my dad constantly fretting, going to work, coming home, making sure me and my sister were OK, feeding us all, visiting my mum as well as maintaining the house at home. It became a very hard time but we got through it, together.

I will never understand my mum's pain, because I obviously haven't experienced it myself, but it hurts me to see her in so much pain. To wake up in the middle of the night having your mum crying out in pain, and having to be rushed to hospital because she can't handle it, is a horrible sight, especially for a young child around the age of 10 or even younger. All I can say is that it scares me to have to watch my mum go through this pain. To also have a chance of developing this disease in my adult years or the idea that I could have to watch my son or daughter go through it as well terrifies me, but I will always see the advantages in life and not let it drag me down.

My points to any young children, whether you're a daughter, son, brother, and sister or any relation to someone who suffers with Crohn's, don't let it get you down. I understand how hard it can be, and I also know it doesn't get any better, especially if it is a close relation, but just keep your head held up high for whoever it may be. Just think you're lucky enough to still have them alive in this world today. Hold their hand and be there for them whenever you can, but also don't let it affect your everyday life. If you have a relative in hospital and you're there sitting at school, channel your sadness, frustration or even anger into your work, it will help matters instead of losing yourself and falling behind in certain subjects.

Also, to any adult or parent suffering with Crohn's disease, don't lie to those around you – such as relatives and children. My mum and dad never lied to me about my mum's illness, which helped, even though we didn't fully comprehend what it was when we were younger, now we're older we understand.

Also don't forget to smile, remember it's contagious."

Raechel

Raechel is the sister of Katie (whose story is above). She's 18 and works as a receptionist. Here is her account of how her mother's Crohn's diagnosis has affected the family.

"Prince Albert, husband of Queen Victoria; Dan O'Bannon, American screenwriter; Dynamo, English magician and Dwight D. Eisenhower, 34th President of the United States - all suffered with Crohn's disease.

My mother suffers with Crohn's disease.

I don't remember a time when my mother wasn't suffering with Crohn's, it's always just been there. Growing up with someone you love, constantly suffering from this disease, isn't easy. I have a very funny feeling that this is a glimpse into parenthood, the constant worrying and caring with the urge to do anything and everything to try and stop the pain, but as with most things, it is an entirely helpless situation.

If I could make a deal with the devil and swap my place with my mother, if I could give my mother my bowel, I would.

I was extraordinarily young when my mother's first symptoms started to develop. She was in and out of hospital frequently. I can remember thinking as a child that something is wrong but not really questioning it, as I would have done now. One night, I remember my father was working (he used to work nights), and my mother was extremely ill. I kept a record of her temperature, when she was sick and when she took medicine. I thought of myself as a doctor, doing what mummy does for me when I'm ill. I remember my dad coming home and telling me I did a good job, looking after mummy.

As a young child, it was different, not knowing what was wrong when your mother was in pain. It wasn't something to be questioned, mummy was just unwell, like when you ate too much chocolate cake and got a tummy ache. It seemed normal at first, just like a cold or something. I don't really remember when I figured out or when I was told that it was something more. Something permanent.

The hospital was my mother's second home, it seemed normal to be there after a while. I can remember being at school and just waiting to leave so I could go and see my mum. It was normal. I can remember having picnics in the summer, and my dad explaining the seasons to me one time after I had questioned him about the sudden abundance of daffodils; the Saturday nights when we would watch Ant and Dec's Saturday Night Takeaway after we had to drive to mum's favourite fish and chip shop and wanting to give mum a specially long hug after we had to leave again, and my sister and father going on ahead to fetch the car, and then yelling at me to hop in the back as he slowly drove away, like the movies.

It all kind of blurs, the good and the bad, and time has practically dissolved from my memories. I remember this one Christmas, this one was bad. It was hard with mum not being there. She was in bed and I can't remember seeing her much that day. All I remember is my dad telling me that mum wasn't well and we had to put our presents in our bedrooms. To me, as a child, being told to organise, tidy and put your presents in your room on Christmas was criminal. Surely this was illegal, it was Christmas, but by now when mum was ill, anything goes. It was just how things were, I suppose.

My mother had major surgery and some of her bowel was removed to try and help with the disease. I don't remember a lot from this time. Looking back, I was sad, confused and hurt about the fact that I couldn't just see my mum, that we never took holidays every year like other children did, and that my mum couldn't enjoy or even come to amusement parks, country walks or even swimming.

After the major surgery, everything seemed to get better. It wasn't as much of a drastic issue. It was still a regular occurrence, but not one that was very disruptive. It became something to laugh about and something to know you've overcome and are stronger because of. One New Year's evening, we had family and friends over and were having a ball welcoming in the new year. We played a game similar to charades, but with the names of every person in the room and you had to act like that person. My uncle Steve got my mum and for his charade, bent over, pretending to be doubled over in pain. I laugh about this every time I think about it, because it's true. My mum wouldn't be my mum if she didn't have her moments.(Her bouts of pain are called "moments" in our house. I'm not sure when or how it started, but it seems to fit). Whenever she had a moment, she would swear in frustration and we'd all jump, scared about what we had done wrong. With me, it was normally stealing her chocolate…

Humour helps. Laughing is a good thing. As a family, we laugh and joke and try to make every sad situation a happy one. One of the funniest stories from when I was a child was when my mother had to have a diabetes test. I was asked by the nurse to help and distract my mother while she administered the test. She turned to me and said: "After 3: 1… 2… 3" and my mind went blank. Distract my mother, how? I don't know what came over me, but before I knew it, my mother had a hand-print on her cheek. I slapped my mother. I had slapped my mother. Everyone around me wore faces of shock. It was one of the funniest memories I have, ever.

It hasn't got any easier since then. It's only gotten harder as I have grown up. The constant worry that my mum is unwell or might need to go back into hospital and that she needs me. I must text or phone my mum every single day, to ask if she is OK. Whenever she has a moment, the worry builds and memories come back from the first time round, and it's hard to push them aside. Selfishly, I also worry about myself – will I have Crohn's? And if I do have Crohn's, will it affect my love life, will I find someone as brave and courageous as my dad, and does it affect pregnancy? How much will it affect my career? How much will it change? How much will it hurt, because my pain threshold is nothing compared to my mother's – she is unbelievably strong.

Personally, I believe that my mother having Crohn's has made us a better family, and me a better person. As a family, we have had to pull together to get through some rather difficult situations. I feel that has made us closer; all the usual "my mother doesn't get me", "I can't talk to my dad because he's my dad" stuff, doesn't matter – I couldn't live without my parents. We can talk about anything and every issue that seems insignificant in comparison to my mother's illness is something I know I can get through with my mum, dad and sister's help.

I have matured and grown up earlier than one should have to. I haven't had the classic teenage rebellion; I couldn't bear to put my parents through any more unnecessary pain. I feel like I have a better understanding of things, which I

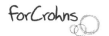

wouldn't have – had it not been for my mum being ill. But I don't think about this much, because this is my normal and I am more than OK with that.

To people like me, who have a parent that suffers with Crohn's: it sucks, doesn't it? People have said to me, that yes, although your life has some misfortune, there are people who have had worse. Well, no matter how much misfortune someone has in their life, you will hate yours. Everyone has misfortune, it's terrible and it can seem all-consuming. Just find whatever way you can to make it better. Whether, like me, you find humour in the darkest of times, or whether you find that reading a good book, or watching films lets you escape. Don't hold on to darkness; find laughter and happiness in whichever way you can.

To parents who are suffering with Crohn's and have young children: don't lie. My parents never lied. Well almost – I still bring up Santa Clause as often as possible. I understand the need to protect them from something big and horrible, but something is going to drastically change in their lives too, not just yours because you've been diagnosed. All I can remember (all I chose to remember) are the picnics we had in hospital gardens, or eating unhealthy food in the family room of the hospital ward, watching Ant and Dec's Saturday Night Takeaway, or pretending to be James Bond in the car when we left the hospital. The bad stuff will stick with you if that's all you have. Good memories wipe away the bad ones. Get the greatest moments out of every day. It's bloody hard, but it's possible. Even the word "impossible" says "I'm possible".

Summary

It can be frustrating for those people closest to Crohn's patients. We naturally want to be able to help those suffering, but often feel helpless. Just being there to listen and support, or with a shoulder to cry on can be a massive help. It is important to understand that sometimes during flare-ups, people with Crohn's may need more sleep, may have to cancel plans and may need time off work or school. As a relative or friend, you can be there to support them and make sure they are getting the rest and affection they need. There are many others out there – people in your situation who also have a loved one suffering from this disease. Finding and talking to these people can be enormously helpful for practical as well as emotional support and advice.

Section 4

What the future holds

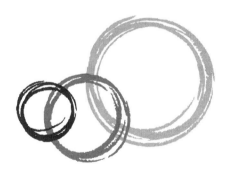

What the future holds

The research interest in Crohn's disease is enormous. Many units throughout the world are investing large sums of money to try and understand Crohn's better, and to produce improved treatments. St Mark's Hospital is one example of a leading institution with a large research interest in inflammatory bowel disease in general, and Crohn's in particular, but there are other large units in the UK and around the world also performing high-quality research in Crohn's disease.

Many of the research projects underway and being published at the moment are interested in the aetiology or pathogenesis of Crohn's – that is, the way in which Crohn's occurs and causes inflammation leading to symptoms and disease. In particular, the genetics of Crohn's, the malfunction of the immune system and the bacteria and other microorganisms which might play a role in causing Crohn's disease. The genetics of Crohn's remains only partially understood and although some very interesting and important genetic markers have been identified for specific aspects of Crohn's, there is relatively little in the way of large-scale genetic 'typing' of Crohn's patients at the moment – although this work is underway in several places. The hope is that a deeper understanding of the genetics of the disease may enable improved treatments and better targeting of particular drugs to patients who are more likely to benefit from them while reducing side-effects.

The immune system is the body's defence against invasion and infection by microorganisms like bacteria and viruses. A malfunction in the immune system is thought to contribute to the inflammation seen in Crohn's disease. Several cells and molecules are under investigation as potential culprits in this inflammation, in the hope that drugs targeting them will be effective in controlling the inflammation, reducing symptoms and producing healing in the diseased areas. Infliximab is a good example of this. It targets a chemical called TNF alpha (which is known to cause inflammation), thereby reducing symptoms and leading to healing in some people. Several other drugs are in the experimental phase of their production, and new evidence will lead to even newer drugs being created in the future.

The role of bacteria and other micro-organisms, or their products, in causing Crohn's is also under investigation by many groups. A deeper understanding of this role may also lead to improved treatments or perhaps protection against harmful agents. There is a great deal of evidence that bacteria in the gut are important in health, and also in influencing inflammation in Crohn's disease. Exactly what form this influence takes, which aspects of the bacteria are responsible, how we can harness the anti-inflammatory properties of some bacteria and nullify the harmful effects of others, is less well understood and is the subject of much debate and research.

There is also lots of work assessing current treatment strategies: improving the types of tests we perform on patients with Crohn's, identifying the impact on quality of life that particular aspects of the disease, treatments or operations have on patients and generally trying to improve the lot of people with Crohn's within the current range of treatments we have. This type of research is also very important, as it helps improve lives *now*, rather than waiting for future drugs to appear which may or may not be effective.

An easy disease would have been cured by now. Crohn's is complex, multi-faceted and cruel. It is also fascinating and full of interesting conundrums and problems. Many brilliant researchers in leading institutions around the world continue to strive to understand Crohn's better, in the hope of helping those with the disease. Progress is frustratingly slow for those who suffer or watch their loved ones do so, but it is made, day by day, and through collaboration between researchers from across the globe, we are significantly closer to a full understanding than we were 10 years ago. Who knows what the next 10 years will bring…

Section 5

Links and further information

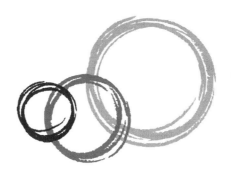

Links and further information

Charities

- forCrohns www.forCrohns.org

- forCrohns buddy system forcrohns.org/site/forcrohns-buddy-system/

- Crohn's & Colitis UK www.crohnsandcolitis.co.uk

- Crohn's in Childhood Research Association (CICRA) www.cicra.org/

- Mind (mental health charity) www.mind.org.uk

Information

- Patient information www.patient.co.uk/health/crohns-disease-leaflet

- British Association for Counselling and Psychotherapy www.bacp.co.uk

- Information for those travelling with Crohn's disease via www.ibdpassport. com

Clinical

- NICE guidance on management of Crohn's disease www.publications.nice. org.uk/crohns-disease-cg152

- IBD Standards

- *A document endorsed by clinical bodies to ensure patients receive consistent high quality care* www.ibdstandards.org.uk/

- British Society of Gastroenterology guidelines for the management of IBD www.bsg.org.uk/clinical-guidelines/ibd/guidelines-for-the-management-of-inflammatory-bowel-disease.html